Saving Delaney

Saving Delaney

From Surrogacy to Family

Andréa AND Keston Ott-Dahl

CLEiS
PRESS

Published in the United States by Cleis Press, an imprint of Start Midnight, LLC, 101 Hudson Street, Thirty-Seventh Floor, Suite 3705, Jersey City, NJ 07302.

Printed in the United States.
Cover design: Scott Idleman/Blink
Cover photograph: Shelley Tosh
Text design: Frank Wiedemann

First Edition.
10 9 8 7 6 5 4 3 2 1

Trade paper ISBN: 978-1-62778-168-8
E-book ISBN: 978-1-62778-169-5

Disclaimer

This is a work of creative nonfiction. Although most texts and emails were transcribed, the conversations in the book all come from the authors' recollections and point of view, though they were not written to represent word-for-word conversations. Rather, the authors have retold them as remembered in a way that evokes the feeling and meaning of what was said, and in all instances, the essence of the dialogue is accurate as perceived by the authors. While all the happenings in this book are true, some names and identifying details have been changed to protect the privacy of certain people involved.

For Andréa, Mom, and Delaney, my warrior women

Andréa, thank you, babe, for being not only my technical writer and fact-checker, but also allowing me to tell the entire story.

Mom, I miss you every day.

Delaney, you are the true hero in this story and my life.
Thank you for being my teacher.

CHAPTER 1

Four Lesbians and a...Baby?

March 3, 2012

THE CLIENTELE THAT NIGHT MADE THE RUN DOWN tavern feel more like an upscale Silicon Valley lesbian nightclub than the San Jose Veterans Hall dive bar that it was. I was thrilled to see so many lesbians at Kris's fortieth birthday bash, although I didn't quite fit in with this chic crowd.

In fact, I stuck out like a sore thumb with my rocker style. My choppy dark shoulder length hair was highlighted with bleach and bright red streaks. I wore thick black eye liner, had my nose pierced and visible tattoos. My holey jeans, tight black vest, boots and gothic jewelry clashed with the well-tailored clothing that most of the guests were wearing.

For a long time, Kris, who was my partner Andréa's cousin, had been the only lesbian she had known. Feeling more at home than at a more formal family setting, this was the perfect venue for Andréa to introduce me to her father's side of the family, and we were excited to be on a kid-free date night. The party was in full swing.

I was especially surprised to see Andréa socializing as I approached her with cocktails in hand. She was in deep conversation with an attractive short woman who was slightly overweight and had long sandy blond hair.

"You aren't going to believe what Erica and her partner Liz have gone through to have a baby," Andréa told me as she brushed wisps of blond hair back from her face. Andréa was stunning as usual, but that night she sparkled in a sexy black dress. Her A-line haircut, short in the back and long in the front, was falling in her face. It made her seem sexy and mysterious and her make-up was perfect. Andréa had the look of a model getting ready to walk down the runway.

The bar was loud and crowded, so I leaned in to hear her more clearly over a group of intoxicated women singing karaoke.

"They've been trying for years," Andréa said, evidently enthralled by the conversation.

I politely smiled but was not thrilled with the topic. *Oh brother!* I thought. The last thing I wanted to talk about was kids, but at least Andréa was being more social. So after handing over her drink, I smiled and held my hand out toward the gal Andréa had been talking to.

"I am Keston," I said, shaking her hand.

"My wife," Andréa proudly interjected. I was sure she was announcing her own coming out, proud as a peacock with her new feathers. Even though we were not legally married, nor was gay marriage available in California at the time, we still called each other "wife," because, for all intents and purposes, that's what we were.

I learned during my brief introduction to Erica that she had dated Andréa's cousin Kris for many years. They had since split up, but still remained good friends. Andréa had grown up thinking of Erica as a cousin, since she was a staple at family holiday events. She was obviously excited to see Erica. It wasn't hard to understand why.

I immediately liked Erica. She was jovial, outgoing, animated, and just a really nice person. She had pale blue eyes that sparkled along with a huge, genuine smile. Unlike the rest of the clientele Erica was dressed plainly with a corduroy tan blazer and generic dark blue jeans. She had the kind of accent you associate with people from New York, and she spoke as much with her hands as she did with her mouth. I could easily imagine Erica as a comedian or as some sort of supporting character starring in comedies.

Unfortunately, just as soon as I got who Erica was, the conversation went right back to children.

Ugh! I grimaced.

"And I have kids now," Andréa beamed as she told Erica.

I politely stood by and faked interest, but easily found my attention drawn behind me as some girl under a blue spotlight in the otherwise dark and dingy bar massacred a karaoke version of Madonna's "Like a Virgin." If you couldn't hear the melody in the background, you would have no idea what song she was singing. Yet I still tried to keep an ear open to the conversation and give an occasional nod to Andréa and Erica's discussion about the kids.

Glancing over my shoulder at the fashionably dressed lesbian at the microphone, a mischievous thought came over me. I knew I was about to make a good impression on Andréa's family. I handed Andréa my drink and then headed off to the dance floor straight to the karaoke DJ. Andréa didn't seem to notice that she now had two drinks in her hands or that I had even left.

Within minutes, I had the entire bar staring at me as I began singing Led Zeppelin's "Whole Lotta Love." That is everyone except Andréa and Erica! I didn't care though; she was not who I was trying to impress this time. As I was belting out the last "ma, ma, ma," I saw Andréa showing pictures to Erica on her cell phone. I assumed it was of her crowning achievements, Jared and Julianna, gorgeous blond spitting images of their beautiful mother.

When I was finished, I casually walked off the dance floor as everyone was clapping, hooting, and hollering their appreciation at me.

Little do they know I have been singing Led Zeppelin tunes with a Janis Joplin twist semi-professionally for years! I thought trying to withhold a snickering smile.

Although I was middle-aged and only five feet tall in heels, this night onstage, I felt like I was twenty again and ten feet tall. This was a great way to break the ice in getting to know Andréa's family.

As I made my way back to Andréa and Erica, family members had clearly warmed up to me as aunts, uncles, and cousins gave me high fives as I walked through the crowd. Feeling rather pleased with myself, I found Andréa and Erica had switched subjects from Jared and Julianna and were now back on the topic of Erica and her partner's infertility dilemma. Having just rocked the room though, I was now in a great mood and was a little more engaged in the conversation.

"So, Erica and Liz have tried everything to have a baby," Andréa repeated as she handed my drink back to me. The two decided they should catch me up on the conversation.

"And we've spent almost a quarter of a million dollars," Erica added.

Wow! I thought, now listening more intently. I had no idea how expensive it was for lesbians to try to make a baby.

"And now they're trying to adopt," Andréa continued.

"But we keep getting turned down. It's hard to adopt when you're *gay*." Erica emphasized the word. "The only country that allows same-sex couples to adopt is the United States," she said as she continued to explain how they couldn't adopt from other countries like straight couples could.

This back-and-forth continued in a heartbreaking way, as I watched with my head bobbing from one direction to the other.

Even though both Erica and Liz were only in their forties, their eggs were bad. Erica said, "We're too old," for them to hope for their own babies. They had tried many times during the past six years, only to have had false pregnancies, miscarriages, and denied adoptions. They had even gone to Stanford for tests and studies. Nothing had worked. Now they were on another waiting list to adopt, and adoption would cost them another forty thousand dollars! Even so, they were likely to be denied babies from birth mothers who, as Erica put it, said they smoked only one pack a day now or had been clean and sober for two weeks— all because they were gay.

"That's terrible," I frowned, shaking my head as Erica went on. Andréa was deeply engrossed in the conversation, nodding and shaking her head sometimes with her mouth gaping open. It appeared that this topic was going to dominate the rest of our evening.

Eventually a striking Middle-Eastern woman swaggered over with a glass of white wine in her hand and kissed Erica on the cheek.

"This is Liz," Erica said as she introduced us to her partner. I was grateful for the interruption.

Liz, who had been celebrating at a different table, shook Andréa's and my hands without much interest. She had a glazed look in her eyes that made me think she'd had a few drinks already and was in celebratory mode. I could relate. I always joke, "I'm an occasional drinker, but occasionally I drink too much!" It looked as if that night was one of those occasions for Liz.

I could tell how different Liz was from Erica. Even though she had an air of confidence, she seemed much more subdued, and my first impression was that she was either shy or just another snob. Although she'd clearly had a few glasses of wine, she maintained a composure that gave me the feeling she had the hidden dominant personality of someone who likes to stay in control. She was also impeccably dressed in a white button down shirt and black slacks. I could tell her appearance was important to her; she had good taste and money.

She seemed to listen a lot and nod or shake her head in approval or disapproval while eying Erica in a way that only couples do. I got the feeling that Liz and Erica were a strong, loving couple as Liz tightly held onto Erica's hand.

Erica and Andréa were still thoroughly involved in chatting about the "baby dilemma." Soon the topic seemed to either bore or tire Liz, much like me. I wondered whether she was sick of reliving the trials and heartbreaks of trying to get pregnant and adopt. It seemed that, as quickly as she could, she excused herself and went back to her friends.

Relief would soon come for me as well when I realized my glass was empty, the perfect reason to excuse myself. "I'm going to get another drink," I told Andréa. "Do you want one?" With all that talking, she wasn't even close to finishing with her first drink. I made my way back to wait in the long line at the bar.

Just as it was my turn to order a drink, I felt someone pressing up against me, hugging my waist with one hand and pushing me up against the bar. I turned and was relieved to see Andréa's beautiful face as she kissed my cheek.

"Good thing that's you," I joked as she put her now-empty glass down in front of me. At that moment, the bartender looked over at me, and I raised two fingers to let him know that I wanted two drinks.

Feeling better now that Andréa had quit the baby dilemma talk, I squeezed her arm around me tighter as she nuzzled my neck, kissing up toward my ear and whispering. But I didn't hear sweet nothings or suggestive compliments. No, Andréa sweetly dropped the mother of all bombshells into my unsuspecting ear.

"I want to surrogate for them," she whispered.

I gasped, "What?" As quickly as my smile had appeared, it was gone in a flash as I jerked my head around to look at her. "No way!" My head was shaking from side to side.

Andréa started pleading. "I feel so bad for them. Here I am with two beautiful babies. I can make babies anytime, and just look what they've gone through, Keston."

"Yeah, it's really sad," I agreed, "But being a *surrogate*? Uh-uh," my head was still shaking.

Her eyes looked so imploring. I told her that we would have to talk about it later. We were still waiting for the bartender to pour our drinks when the next thing I knew, Erica and Liz came up behind us.

I was beginning to get scared. The way Erica and Andréa had reconnected so quickly made me think that Andréa might have already blurted out to Erica that she would consider surrogating. It was obvious that the two had wanted this new evolution in the conversation to continue and Erica had gone to bring in Liz, who was now much more interested in us.

What the hell is happening? I thought.

We finally got our drinks and moved to the other side of the bar.

"Are you serious?" Erica asked Andréa point-blank.

"Yes," Andréa replied without hesitation.

So much for our talking about it, I frowned.

"Well, if you're serious, we'd definitely be interested," Erica said directly.

Excitement was building between Andréa, Erica, and now Liz. "Your kids are so beautiful!" Erica continued.

Liz now nodded while intently looking at Andréa as if she were trying to read her.

"Hold on, slow down," I kept saying over and over, putting my hand down on an imaginary table between the women. But it was no use—the three were unstoppable.

Erica sweetened the deal: "Of course, we'll pay you."

Andréa wasn't working at the time, since the cost of daycare outweighed what monies she would bring in, and she felt ashamed about it. Now Andréa got a big smile as she looked at me persuasively with Erica's sweetening of the deal. "Babe, it would be like a job for me; I can contribute to the family." Erica's eyes grew wider as she nodded, looking directly at me with Liz still nodding behind her.

I felt like I was in a used-car sales lot being tag-teamed by Andréa and Erica.

"Wait a minute," I said to the three and pulled Andréa off to the side.

"Andréa, I was through raising my kids when we started dating; now I have at least another fourteen years and have taken on raising Jared and Julianna. I can't do this," I shook my head.

"Babe, this isn't *our* baby. We will not be raising this baby. I will only be making it to hand off to them," Andréa pleaded her case as she dragged me back toward Liz and Erica.

Liz let Erica do the talking and didn't say much herself, but she inserted "uh-huh"s and "yes"es from time to time, with a growing smile on her face.

I realized having a child was a dream for both of these women, not just Erica, and I did feel bad for them, but this was all going way too fast.

"Panda, we have to talk about it when we get home. This means a whole year out of our lives," I said, speaking to Andréa but looking intently at each of the three women. I definitely wanted Liz and Erica to know that I was not going to give my blessing right then and there. This wasn't something to be decided so quickly. I needed to get Andréa out of there.

Andréa and I had booked a room at an Embassy Suites for the night. We'd planned to leave the party early to spend time together without the kids. "We should get going. We have *plans*," I reminded her. Luckily, Andréa loves our romantic time, so she took no convincing. We quickly excused ourselves after Andréa and Erica traded contact information and then said goodbye to the rest of the family.

I had an anxious feeling as we left the San Jose Veterans Hall that night. Knowing Andréa, I could tell she was serious and would not let go of the idea of being a surrogate. I wasn't worried that she couldn't give the baby up at the end. I knew that she was the rare type of woman who could, to the right people. I was worried about what a pregnancy would mean to our relationship and the little freedom we already had.

After all, it was only a year and a half since my mother's death. Subsequently, I'd had a mini nervous breakdown and pushed every responsibility out of my life so that I could live carefree. Gradually my plan had been spiraling out of control, and I was gaining more responsibility than I could ever imagine.

Little did I know at the time that we had just stepped onto the biggest life-changing roller coaster of our lives.

How did I get here? I thought, unaware of what was about to happen. *Mom would have been horrified.*

CHAPTER 2

Mom and Her Shadow

MOM WOULD HAVE SEEN NO REASON TO HELP THESE women, let alone give them a baby.

My mother's life wasn't easy. Shirley Ann Spiers was born in 1925. Her parents were poor and often relied on the kindness of strangers to get by. Growing up during the hard times of the Great Depression shaped who Mom became, a no-nonsense woman. In her teens, she felt it was her duty to join the efforts in World War II and became a WAVE in the navy. To say she loved America would be an understatement. She always supported her country and the president. If the president was a Democrat, she was a Democrat. If he was Republican, she was Republican. She was patriotic until the day she died.

After the war, she moved to southern California to become a starlet. She was as beautiful as Grace Kelly and had Golden Girl Dorothy Zbornak's snide, snarky humor.

Every man chased Mom. She was very witty, thin, petite, stunningly beautiful, and could make throwing back a shot of Scotch while she smoked a cigar look sexy and feminine as she teased her pearl necklace with perfectly manicured fingernails. Her strength and beauty must have been intoxicating to men—too intoxicating. Eventually several failed marriages left her a single mom from the mid-1950s through the late 1970s, raising five children without a penny of child support. She had to give up her dreams. Often she had to make hard decisions to keep her family afloat when the going got tough.

She was forty-one years old and in the process of divorcing my father by the time she had me, the baby of five kids. Even though I was a tomboy, I was a petite blond version of her, and her shadow. I admired everything about her.

While my mother was a strong woman, she was definitely not one-dimensional. Just like anyone else, she had flaws. My awe of her made it hard for me to see them, but she was human. It was painfully obvious how cold Mom was to her oldest children, my two older sisters, Rhonda and Lindsay. After they grew up and moved out of the house, they were not close with Mom, and besides annual birthday cards and Christmas Eve, Mom did not attempt to make much contact with them. Rhonda was married and pregnant by the time I was born—we rarely saw her—and Lindsay was a handful for Mom. She was raised in the free-loving Sixties. Complete with long, flowing hair and bell-bottom jeans, Lindsay embraced hippie living at a young age. She ran away often, immersed herself in drugs, and more than once got pregnant as a teenager. By the mid-Seventies, though, abortion was legal, and from what I understand, Mom gave Lindsay no other choice than to abort the pregnancies. I'm not sure either of them ever quite forgave the other. They became more estranged as Lindsay grew up.

Admittedly, one of Mom's not-so-wonderful traits was that she was a bigot. She had not been exposed to diversity the way we are today. She had no idea that she had prejudices. She would say, "Of course I don't treat or think of those people any differently," not realizing that calling them "those people" was prejudice. I don't think she ever knew an African-American person, let alone had one as a friend or even an acquaintance. She made a big deal once of befriending a Mexican man she worked with because he spoke "beautifully." She had another female friend at work who had a mentally disabled son, and she told me (not in a gossipy tone, but more as a matter of disgusted sympathy for her friend), "You know her son is an imbecile."

Needless to say, I grew up emulating Mom. She was my closest friend and confidant even when I was a teen. Out of her five children I was most like her and I always had the impression she lived vicariously through me.

Unfortunately, though, I was a little too much like Mom. I made bad choices that disappointed her at times, even though they were some of the same choices she had made at that age. Like Mom, I had been married, divorced and was a single mother by the time I was twenty. As I think back on it, perhaps I made those same mistakes subconsciously in my quest to emulate her.

But she always quickly rallied behind me. I also didn't realize it, but like Mom, I had also formed my own bigotries.

Real-Life Monsters

I loved to drive the southern California highways as if I were racing at Daytona Beach, weaving in and out of traffic at ninety miles per hour. I had no concern for my safety (or anyone else's). When I was twenty-five, the California penal system had had enough of my freeway shenanigans. After I spent a few days in jail, a kind judge felt I could use some good old community service. I was sentenced to work ten days at a state facility for disabled adults in Anaheim.

The place was a one-story building, run-down, dirty, and with long, dingy-yellow halls that used to be white. The second I walked through the doors, I was hit by a repulsive odor. The place reeked of cleaning agents, feces, and bad cooking all mixed together. The charge nurse immediately led me to the laundry room at the back of the building. There I got the lucky assignment of washing, drying, and folding the patients' clothes. I spent the next ten days, eight hours per day, reaching into huge vats of laundry soaked with urine and shit.

The patients there had cerebral palsy, Down syndrome, or other disabilities. I lumped all of them into one "retarded" category in my terrified mind. Each day on my way through the hallway to the laundry room, I saw people in wheelchairs who were wearing helmets, drooling all over themselves, or sitting in their own excrement. After my eight-hour shift was over, I often passed the same people in that hallway, still sitting in their excrement. Even though I was pretending not to notice them, I could smell them as I walked by as fast as I could to get myself away from them, horrified they might approach or touch me.

Occasionally, one of those lonely patients would come wandering back to the laundry room, wanting some form of human interaction. I quickly learned to hide behind the big door, or else I might be subjected to kisses or have someone try to hold my hand before a nurse finally came around looking for him or her.

I felt sickened by the residents of the facility, afraid of them, and very sad. They were not well taken care of by the overworked staff, and I never once saw a family member visiting. *Why does God allow this?* I wondered in despair every day as I left. I thought that these "imbeciles" were obviously the inspirations for monsters in horror films like *Frankenstein*. And they were my punishment for my misdeeds to society.

I was deeply affected, and not in a positive way. Once my community service was over, I got as far away as I could. Afterward I did my best to suppress memories of that place and those people, although at times they would pop up and haunt me. But I never talked about it to anyone, and I never, ever drove the California highways like an idiot again.

Emerging from Her Shadow

When Mom was in her mid-Sixties, she had a brain aneurysm that almost killed her. Overnight she permanently retired, and I became the reluctant matriarch of the family. Since we were so much alike and so close, it was a natural progression. Obviously, I would end up taking care of her. But she wasn't helpless, and she would help me by taking care of my kids while I worked (and partied).

In the Eighties, at just nineteen, I gave up my dream of pursuing an acting career when I had a daughter, whom I named Jordan, and whom Mom helped me raise. At twenty-seven, I had my son Zack and was much more mature and prepared to be a parent. He and I would end up having a similar relationship as the one I had with Mom. He was born with an old soul, very wise and thoughtful. When he was young, we spent countless hours having deep conversations about our goals, what he could be in life.

After two failed marriages, I realized I was gay, but since I was already well into my thirties, it just wasn't that big a deal. I did have an epiphany, like most gay people do, but times were different, and I didn't really care what anyone thought; it was none of their business. Mom realized it—I never told her, but she told me.

One night when I was picking up the kids, Mom blurted out just as I was walking out the door, "By the way, I know you are that way. And I don't care. I love you no matter what." She sounded proud of herself. She was delighted after that when I brought home attractive women for her to meet. Mom would whisper to me in a surprised tone, "She's pretty!" Nodding approval with a raised eyebrow.

"Of course, Ma. What did you think, I would bring home an ugly woman for you to meet?" I joked with her.

"Well, I thought, you know," Mom paused, "You're feminine, and so I thought you'd bring home a manly girl. I mean, isn't that how it is for *you* people?" She had stereotypically assumed I would bring home girls with crew cuts, plaid flannel shirts, and Birkenstock sandals.

I smiled, adoring her naïveté.

"Oh, things are different now, Ma. As a matter of fact, if being gay were more accepted in your time, I think you would have probably met Ms. Right instead of all those Mr. Wrongs!"

She thought about it for a few seconds. "You know, maybe you're right," she nodded.

It was not long at all after I came out that I became popular in the lesbian crowd. I was a self-proclaimed "queen bee." My annual parties were well known, and I was always taking off on some fantastic, adventurous lesbian weekend while Jordan and Zack stayed with Mom, until they were old enough to take care of themselves.

Somewhere along the way, I also became the friend of the friendless. I was well known for befriending some of the lonelier gals, inviting them to my parties or along on my adventures so they could make more friends. That was unique for queen bees, and oftentimes caused cattiness among some of the other popular women in the community who were less welcoming. They snickered at my loner pals and how they dressed, with their tattoos and piercings. For some reason, I related to outcasts.

Mom and I both got older, and she began having more serious health issues. Her five-foot-four stature gradually shrank to less than my five feet. She had a wheelchair, which she barely used because she "wouldn't be caught dead in that thing," but as the years went by, she started using it more and more. It broke my heart to see her decline, and in taking care of her, I became much softer and more thoughtful.

Along with cold decision-making, without knowing, she taught me lessons of humanity. Little did we know how those lessons would affect both of us.

CHAPTER 3

My Coldest Decision

October 29, 2010

This time it feels different.

"This is it," I said, thinking aloud to myself as I parked my Ford Explorer in the hospital emergency room parking lot. Then a quick smile came over me as I realized how many other times I had thought that before.

I had always imagined that I would find Mom dead in her bed when I came to visit. Often I would call her, and when she didn't answer the phone, I'd drive the twenty minutes to her apartment in ten, only to find her watching *Jeopardy* with the TV on so loud, she couldn't hear the phone. I hoped she would have a peaceful death; after all, she was eighty-four.

Mom was now only sixty-seven pounds, but she still had beautiful long white hair, which had been dark brown. This was her seventh trek to the hospital in eight years for pneumonia; she was a tough old bird, and I was her champion. Together we pulled her through some

amazing, unbeatable odds despite the many doctors' typical predic-
tions of her imminent death. Her strong will and my knowledge about
her COPD, a chronic obstructive pulmonary disease that causes severe
difficulty in breathing, made us an unstoppable team.

She was still as sharp as a tack, usually flirting with the doctors and
putting on lipstick through her gasps for air. Miss Shirley Ann Spiers
had outlived both her parents and most of her friends, despite the fact
that she'd smoked since she was fifteen years old and drank like a fish.
Although, as classy as she always was, I'd never seen her sloppy.

I met the ambulance drivers who brought Mom in for respiratory
distress in triage and held Mom's hand as I answered intake questions
from the nurse. This was routine for us, except this time Mom was not
flirting or smiling as she usually did. She seemed dazed and unusually
quiet as the middle-aged male ER doctor on duty evaluated her. He was
pudgy, with thinning hair.

He looked over at me the same way they always did, as if to say,
you know this is bad, right? Then he said something I wasn't used to
hearing: "I feel like I'm looking at someone who's already going into
rigor mortis, but is still breathing." He added, "Barely breathing."

It was hard for me to take any doctors seriously though. They always
said she wouldn't come out of the hospital.

I chuckled inside. *You do not know my mother, and you do not know her
fear of death!*

In the days that followed, I saw that Mom was in fact different this
time. I had learned long ago not to leave her side very often when she
was in the hospital. I had on more occasions than I cared to remember
found the nurses giving Mom wrong medications or ones that didn't
mix, or sedating her unnecessarily. In the past, I had even lost jobs to
be at Mom's bedside, but jobs could come and go. I knew Mom would
eventually have to leave me, so I let the jobs go instead of putting up
with thoughtless bosses who cared only about sales, not people.

We spent most of the time talking or working on crossword puzzles
during her hospital trips. The time was priceless for me. I learned
so much about her during our deep conversations while she was on

her multiple deathbeds, but this time she was quiet, struggling when she did talk and not preoccupied with her hair and makeup.

After a few days, the steroids and breathing treatments were working, but Mom just seemed more out of it. She would look over at me and smile. I smiled back as I tried to hide my tears so she wouldn't see, as she faded in and out of consciousness, which was unusual.

At nine o'clock in the morning on the fourth day, an attractive dark-haired female doctor on call came in and said, "Can I talk to you?" Mom had had a rough night. Her breathing had become so shallow that they had put her on a CPAP breathing mask to force air into her lungs. She had been on it many times before. Twice in the past, when there was a sudden decline in her breathing she had been intubated and I figured we were going to talk about what steps we would take next.

"Of course," I said, and followed her into the hallway.

She didn't mince words, but I could tell by the sad look on her face that she was a caring woman. "I don't think your mom has long. Her breathing is so shallow. If it were my mother, I would let her go."

"She is afraid," I mumbled as the doctor continued.

She put her hand on my shoulder and said, "She is suffering." The doctor looked at me sympathetically. I was stunned. It was as if she knew how Mom and I had worked so hard over the years to keep her alive.

She looked me in the eye and said, as if she herself were about to cry, "If I take her off the CPAP and oxygen, she'll be gone in just an hour or two." She hesitated and then continued as I stared at her. "I can have you in charge of giving her morphine to make it more peaceful for her."

This time, tears fell down my face as I contemplated "giving up" for the first time. Everything Mom and I did, we did as a team. I wasn't going to make this decision without discussing it with her. "That's up to my mom. Let me talk to her," I told the doctor. I wiped away my tears and went back into the room.

Mom was awake and looked over at me without saying a word. She seemed so tired.

"Mom?" I moved the CPAP breathing mask, which she hated, off her face and sat next to her, leaning close as I held her hand. "Mom, I'm not sure you're going to pull through this time."

Her eyes grew big, and without a word, she gave me a wild "You are out of your mind; of course I am" look. I hesitated, trying to think of what to say.

"Mom, you know you're going to have to go, right?" I said to her in a squeaky voice.

Mom shook her head and whispered through gasps for air, "But where would I go?"

"You will go with Grandpa and Grandma, and your favorite dog Scarlett," I told her. "Aren't you tired, Ma?" I could no longer hold back my tears. "Ma, you have to go now."

Mom lifted her head off the pillow and although gasping for air, she spoke more clearly than before: "The hell with you. I will get up and be out of here like I always do." Then her head dropped back down. It was the first complete sentence I had heard her say in over three days.

I just sat there for a few moments and stared at this warrior woman, my hero, who was barely breathing. She was suffering, and I was suffering. We had done this dance for years now; I knew she had to be tired, because I was tired. But Mom couldn't give up, and it broke my heart to tell her she should; she always needed to see me fighting for her, not against her. But I knew this time was different.

"Okay, Ma. Let me talk to the doctor and see what she says," I said, putting the mask back on her face and bowing my head. Then I got up and walked out the door. But I didn't go to find the doctor. I leaned up against the wall and cried. After about ten minutes, I finally found the doctor sitting at a desk at the nurses' station. She was typing away. I walked over to the desk and got her attention.

"Can you please take my mom off the breathing machine, but first start giving her the morphine?" I asked the doctor.

She gave me nod and a sympathetic crooked smile and said, "Of course."

I didn't feel like I was doing the right thing, but I felt like I was doing what had to be done. I turned around and walked back to Mom's room, but before I entered, I fanned my eyes to dry my tears, took a deep breath, and prepared mentally for the performance of my life.

Mom was barely awake.

"Okay, Mom, we're going to fight!" I smiled and squeezed her hand. She smiled back at me and nodded. "I'm going to fight with you this one last time, Ma. But the doctor said that these machines are not helping you. She says you need to get rest. You have to sleep this off like you have in the past. You have to go to sleep." I spoke directly into her ear.

She nodded without any expression and weakly said, "Okay."

I called my brothers in Texas. Then I texted my sister Lindsay and my daughter Jordan, who lived nearby. I told them they wouldn't make it in time, but gave them the option to come to the hospital. Lindsay was not close to Mom, and if she came, I knew she was coming to support me, not to say goodbye to our mother. I couldn't wait for them or I might change my mind. I might be a coward. This was my burden, and I didn't want to weigh them down with it.

I was on the phone with my boss when the nurse came into the room to start administering morphine into Mom's IV. A few minutes later, the same nurse came in and she started to turn off the machines. She left all the wires hooked up to the overhead monitor, but turned the monitor off. Mom went into a thrashing sleep, which I didn't expect.

"It happens sometimes," the nurse explained. "It can be a side effect of the morphine."

Hours went by. Lindsay arrived, as did Jordan, and we three sat in silence watching Mom's distressed breathing and shaking head. I held her hand the entire time. Each hour I asked the nurses to give her more morphine, and then more, and then again more. Like her many death-beds, Mom took many "last breaths." There were many times when the pause between them made us all think she was gone, only to be shocked when she took another.

More hours went by. Mom was just not giving up. I admired her.

At one point, she opened her eyes and held her hands out, as if she were looking at someone at the foot of her bed. Then her arms flopped back down. Her breathing was even more horrific to watch. She was struggling.

At 8:00 p.m., a new nurse came in, and I said without any inflection in my voice, "Please give my mom some more morphine."

"Of course," the nurse said as she looked at a chart that was hooked to Mom's IV. "You want more morphine?" she asked in a concerned voice.

"Yes, she's struggling," I said.

She hesitated, staring at me, then looked over at Lindsay, then back down at the morphine chart. "We've given her enough morphine to put down a horse. Are you sure?"

"Yes," I said, staring down at the floor.

The nurse politely said, "I'll be right back." I watched her as she walked out, and I could see her pick up the phone at the nurses' station. She soon hung up and came directly to Mom's room. She nodded to me and administered more morphine into the IV.

Mom soon took her last breath at 8:30 p.m. I realized this was it, and with tears pouring down my face, I yelled out, hoping she could hear me, "Thank you, Mom. You were a great mother. If I could be half the woman you were, I would be proud, Ma. I love you!"

Lindsay, Jordan, and I then sat in silence. I still held Mom's hand when all of a sudden, just over my head, the cables still attached to the monitor lifted up—then dropped back down. The three of us gasped!

"What the hell was that?" I said, looking at Lindsay, whose hands were covering her open mouth in shock. She was speechless.

"Did we all just see that?" I asked.

"Yes," Jordan nodded.

Lindsay started to giggle. "That was Mom," she was finally able to blurt out.

I knew in that minute that Mom would always be around, just in a different capacity; I knew she was there. It comforted me. She was going to stay near.

Many people would consider my role in my mother's death humane. I do not feel that way. That day and night, I was the life-or-death decision-maker for someone whom I loved, maybe more than anyone. I played the roles of judge (in giving the verdict that Mom's time was up), jury (in deciding her fate), and executioner (in taking the initiative to make that fate happen). My guilt was overwhelming.

My only solace was that I knew if Mom were in my shoes, she would have made the same decision I had made for her, only she would not have felt guilty about it. She would have been matter of fact about it; it was something that had to be done.

And I also knew that if I had to make that decision over, I would do it again.

A strange feeling swept over me as I walked out of the hospital for the last time. For the first time in more than twenty years, I had no one but myself to take care of. My daughter Jordan had her own life with her fiancé, whom she planned to live with. My son Zack was seventeen going on thirty and had his own plans that no longer included me in his daily life. And now Mom was gone.

At least it's over. I would never be in that position again. But in less than two short years, I was in fact in that position again—in the most unimaginable way.

Death of a Salesman

In the hours, days, and months that followed my mother's death, I started spiraling into a midlife crisis of sorts. I locked away the pain and guilt for my trickery in Mom's death. I went back to being the positive, enthusiastic person I normally was, pretending that my world had not just spun upside down and everything in it had not abruptly changed. I was still in control.

I am free now, I thought, experiencing an unexpected sense of relief. I would free myself even further. Some would say I was on a mission to sabotage my life, but I knew better. My plan was to make my life much less stressful. The very night Mom died, I immediately and coldly went home and told my partner of nine years that I was leaving our lovely but passionless relationship without much more of an explanation. I also informed her that I was not interested in saving our house, as we were more than $260,000 underwater, with a heavy $2,600-a-month mortgage payment. No kids, no mother, no partner, no huge house payment to be responsible for, and now the only other heavy thing on my shoulders was my relentlessly high-pressure job selling architectural signs. Driving home the night Mom died, I knew that one of the first changes I would make was to leave that terrible job—and not just that company. I never wanted to get into a high-pressure, straight-commission sales job again.

I had a little money set aside, and I was going to take time off and enjoy my newfound freedom from everything.

Cougar, Cougar Chaser, or Cougar Catcher?

Andréa and I met at a party shortly after Mom passed. I was the lead singer in a rock cover band, Beautiful Chaos, and that night we were playing at a friend's house party. I was busy entertaining and drinking a never-ending supply of tequila shots handed to us after each song.

The party was at a ranch-style home in an upscale neighborhood in the hills of Walnut Creek. About fifty women were there, along with music and a barbeque. Some of the women were just sitting around listening to the music, and some were playing basketball in the oddly placed court located smack in the middle of the front yard.

Andréa came late. Even though I was in full swing belting out "Piece of My Heart," I, like everyone else, noticed the beautiful, tall blond who had suddenly appeared out of nowhere. She made her way through the crowd and quietly sat in a corner next to a sporty-looking gal. It looked like she was on an informal date with this woman, who wasn't paying much attention to her.

As the party died down, most of the partygoers left, and the remaining diehards were congregating in the kitchen. Andréa was standing there all by herself, looking awkward. She appeared to be in need of rescuing! I thought that perhaps she was an outcast as well. I decided to introduce myself and find out what her story was.

"Hey, why are you standing here all alone?" I asked her.

"No one wants to talk to me," she answered.

"That's hard to believe," I smiled at her. I didn't want to walk away and leave her all alone again, so I continued the conversation.

"What's your story? Who are you here with?" I asked.

I could tell she was shy. I had to ask her a lot of questions to get her to talk. I found out her name was Andréa and that she pronounced it the French way: "On-*dray*-uh." She was twenty-eight years old, a single mother, and didn't get out very often. This was something we had in common, since I had done the single-mom gig for years. Though I could tell she liked talking to me, I thought it was because I was the only one brave enough to approach her. That surprised me; she was so beautiful, but lesbians are a finicky breed.

Eventually I had to leave and join the rest of my band to start loading the truck.

I thought nothing more of our meeting. After all, there was a sixteen-year age difference. Andréa was just one of the many girls I met that night. The next morning, I logged onto my laptop and saw that I had several friend requests on my Facebook page from girls I'd met the night before. Andréa was one of them.

Now, why would a young hottie want to be friends with a middle-aged forty-four-year-old wild child like me? I was puzzled, but I accepted her request.

Instantly after I had confirmed it, I heard a ping. Andréa messaged me. She didn't seem remotely as shy online as she'd been at the party. Soon she got my phone number, and we started texting. By the tone of her texts, I could tell she had a crush on me.

"Someone told me your guitar player used to be your wife," she texted.

"Yep, that is true," I texted back.

"You are too hot for her."

Uh-oh! I thought, but was amused at her flirting. I smiled, and we continued texting over the next few weeks. We talked a lot about her children, Jared and Julianna. Jared was four years old and Julianna was just two.

I kept her flirting at bay, and she didn't push it. I didn't want to lead her on. Having a new, young girlfriend with two children was not on my simple-life plan. I was in a very selfish period. My only priorities were: Where is the next party? Who is going to be there? And what will be my cocktail of choice?

I thought I would just be friends with Andréa, and I planned to help her meet other women, closer to her own age. But Andréa had other plans. She soon let me know I had very little choice in the matter. One night when I took her out to a club to meet other women, she put her secret plans into action. Before I knew what was coming, she had me pinned up against a wall and was kissing me. I couldn't resist her; who could? So I thought we would just have some casual fun, since thoughts of our age difference and her two small children were looming over me.

During a phone conversation, Andréa told me, "You will be the youngest person I've ever seriously dated."

She told me about a relationship that began when she was just eighteen with a thirty-eight-year-old male friend of her parents. She'd grown up knowing him as an informal "uncle" since she was thirteen. The day he first met her, he called her a "hottie," and only a few years later started sending her provocative emails. She thought he was just joking. One day after a family barbecue, he arranged to meet the young and broke teenage Andréa at a gas station, offering to fill up her tank. When giving her a hug goodbye, he surprised her by leaning in and French-kissing her. "Then I realized he wasn't joking," she told me. "I was grossed out. But I was also flattered. Here was this worldly, wealthy older man pursuing me."

He started meeting her at restaurants. Four-hundred-dollar dinners and two-hundred-dollar bottles of wine were intoxicating for a naïve young teenager. Andréa wanted so desperately to protect the "uncle" that she deliberately allowed herself to be seen as a teenage sex kitten who pursued this older, wealthy man and family friend, when nothing could have been further from the truth—at least, it hadn't started that way. It put a further strain on her relationship with some of her family members.

They had dated for four years before she realized that her "uncle" would never tell her he loved her and would never marry her. Feeling unworthy and used, she left him.

Desperate for love and approval, she felt worthless, so she settled on the ex-con drunkard who became the father of her two children only six months after her breakup with the older man.

Her new husband was even older, and very uneducated, but perfect for her at the time, because all she wanted was babies. "Babies would love her forever," she explained to me her mentality at the time. The drunken new husband had already fathered four children with various women, and was more than happy to oblige. After a few years of domestic violence, Andréa finally left him. Apart from the inconsistent fifty dollars a month in child support that he paid for both Jared and Julianna combined, and an occasional phone call to them, while really trying to talk to Andréa, he had taken no responsibility for the children and made no effort to see them.

She had previously had brief relationships with women and found that she was much more emotionally attached to them than to the men she had known. But she was afraid of the stigma that came with being gay. She eventually got tired of hiding in the closet and finally decided to stop faking who she was. With two small children, Andréa dared to come out just a year before we met and begin her life all over again.

Hearing Andréa's past was a lot for me to take in. If I wasn't apprehensive before, I certainly was now. But she was both adorable and persuasive. And, man, she loved me.

Trying to make light of our age difference, Andréa joked, "You see? You're not a cougar chasing younger women," She snickered with a devious smile. "It's me, I'm a cougar chaser." Then she laughed and added, "I mean cougar *catcher*," emphasizing the word.

She was absolutely sure that I was the one. "I just knew from the minute I met you," she told me. "It's different from anything I've ever felt before."

I was unsure and proceeding cautiously. It was impossible to resist the attention and adoration she was giving me. Her confidence in us—in me—was what I initially fell in love with.

Andréa got a job working as an office manager for a gastroenterologist. Before taxes, she was earning $416 a week—and daycare cost her $320. The doctor had her driving all over the East Bay to his various satellite offices. After the cost of gas, the job was costing her more money than she was making, and the doctor didn't even provide health insurance. It made no sense.

I was very concerned that her kids didn't have health insurance. "You need to get help from the state until Julianna is old enough to go to school," I said. "You're a perfect example of why we have state aid."

Andréa was hesitant. "The stigma that comes with it…it's unbearable," she said. "My family will look down on me." She was too proud to apply. But after she lost her job with the doctor, she had no choice. She started counting the years until she could work again, when Julianna would be old enough to be in school and daycare wouldn't eat up her entire paycheck.

I was seeing Andréa and her kids on weekends, and the four of us grew closer and closer.

It wasn't long before I realized that she was much more mature than most of the women I had dated, and that there was far more to Andréa than met the eye.

There's Something about Andréa

Andréa is fifty percent Swiss and twenty-five percent Korean. Her Swiss genes clearly predominate, with her height and blond hair, but if you know she's part Korean and are looking for it, you can see it in her almond-shaped eyes. She's very feminine, but can also "boy up" with a backward baseball cap, tank top, and men's shorts. Andréa doesn't drink alcohol much, and she takes very good care of herself.

In the lesbian world, just like the rest of the world, there are some girls who are just meanies, who have some inherent chip on their shoulder. Before I dated Andréa, I had a brief affair with a meanie. This woman was my own age. I warned her that I had recently had breast-reduction surgery and that my breasts had scars. When we started to become more intimate, she took one look and yelled (yes, yelled!) "Gross! Why would you do that? Why would you mutilate your breasts like that?" Then she gave a big sigh and muttered "Yuck."

Now, why I continued to date this woman is beyond me, but I did for a short while. I knew my scars would slowly disappear, and I was very happy that I had had the procedure done; being five feet tall with breasts that were falling out of a double-D bra had made me look awkward and out of proportion.

A few months later, the meanie and I parted company. I had had a touch-up surgery on my breasts and was wrapped up in surgical tape. It never dawned on me to remove it. I never imagined I would end up getting close to Andréa the night she pinned me to the wall.

We had a great time, and before I knew it, Andréa was having her way with me. She may be shy, but when she wants something, she isn't afraid of going after it. I had completely forgotten that I had the tape still wrapped around my breasts. Andréa took off my shirt and bra, and saw the bandages. She just questioned softly, "Oh?"

I was embarrassed. "Oh, shit, I'm sorry; I forgot about that. Let me go to the bathroom and take that stuff off."

"No, I'll do it." And without giving me time to protest, she began gently pulling off the surgical tape and kissing each inch of my scars as she removed it, not in a sexual way, but in a very loving way.

What a huge difference between these two intimate experiences!

Obviously, it was not hard to fall in love with Andréa. In the beginning, she was hypersexual, but I felt like that persona was an act. She seemed to be the shy secret-sex-kitten girl everyone would want to date. But that wasn't the real Andréa. As soon as I broke through that façade, I realized how much more there was to her. She was even more awkwardly shy than I had thought, though she was never that way with me. I saw a very intelligent person with a good heart.

She was not at all the bimbo she thought everyone wanted.

In my experience, it's rare to find the whole package. That's what Andréa was. I let her know right away that she didn't have to put on that sexy persona for me to love her. I think she was a little surprised, but relieved that she no longer had to perform.

Keeping Life Simple, or Not

I was used to asking Mom for advice, but now she was gone. I began channeling her, imagining what she would say. But soon after Andréa and I started seriously dating, I began to have the nagging feeling it was the other way around, as if Mom was the one channeling me. It felt almost like she was tapping me on the shoulder.

One morning, I woke up very tired. Andréa and I had stayed up late the night before talking. We'd developed a ritual of lying in bed and talking for at least an hour or two before we actually fell asleep.

That morning I was late for an appointment, which was odd for me. I had always been a stickler for being on time. As I was rushing down the stairs thinking about Andréa, I felt a looming presence standing at the bottom. It was Mom. Her presence was so strong, I could almost see her standing there leaning against the end of the banister.

"Are you out of your mind?" she asked me, shaking her head and laughing. *"Aren't you a little old to be playing house?"* I could feel her looking at me as I rushed around searching for my keys.

I tried to ignore her.

"Are you going through a midlife crisis?" she continued.

"I know, Ma. It probably won't be serious. Don't worry," I mumbled. *"Aha! Here they are."* I had located my keys in a basket behind the television and hurried past the imaginary apparition of my mother and toward the door.

Mom didn't give up.

"I'm gone now, Kes. You don't have to take care of anyone but yourself. Aren't you through raising babies? You'll have to take care of all of them, you

know. Why don't you enjoy the rest of your life?" I could hear Mom yell as I closed and locked the door.

She would have thought I had gone insane.

Before I knew it, within only a few months, Andréa and her two beautiful kids, who looked like mini clones of their mother, had moved in with me and Zack (who was rarely home) and my poor, patient ex-wife (who was losing her patience) in my house in northern California while it was in foreclosure. It was a two-story 1980s suburban home built in an upper-middle-class neighborhood. Things were wonderful for Andréa and me, but our living situation wasn't good, to say the least. I know it was awful for my unfortunate ex-wife.

It wasn't long after I started dating Andréa that I noticed my large circle of friends was becoming smaller, and my band broke up. My friends disapproved of my dating someone so much younger, or it was her kids (after all, kids do not go over well in the lesbian party atmosphere), or perhaps their loyalties were with my ex-wife. Whatever it was, I was so busy and absorbed in our life together that I hardly noticed. We did get babysitters at least twice a month so we could get out enough for me to be happy. It was all I needed.

Andréa preferred not to have many friends. "They always let you down," she told me, which I said was cynical and sad. I thought it odd that she wanted to be with someone like me, who had so many friends, when she felt just the opposite.

Within a year, we began looking and finally found our own house, a hundred-year-old Craftsman by the Antioch Marina and the California Delta. It needed a lot of work, but it had two bedrooms upstairs and a huge basement, which I fell in love with. The basement looked like something you would see in a Stephen King horror movie, with a long sea-foam-green hallway that led to four small bedrooms and three bizarre kitchens. (Yes, three kitchens!) The rooms were filled with spider-webbed baby cribs, boxes that looked like they had been there for years, old furniture, and an antique wheelchair. I could only guess that at one point the house had been some sort of speakeasy or boardinghouse. The kitchen upstairs hadn't been remodeled since the 1960s, and the carpeting was horribly stained. Beneath the mess, though, it was our dream house, with all the original built-in wooden hutches and Craftsman-style columns; even the glass in the cabinets was from the early nineteen hundreds. I quickly imagined Zack being able to live downstairs with his college buddies so I could still have him nearby, and he would have his own private door and apartment. Then I saw putting in stairs to the basement from upstairs to make more room for our living quarters. Fixing it up together would be a fun project for Andréa and me.

I had some money set aside, but I couldn't get a mortgage without an income. Andréa and her father Boppi (Swiss for "Dad") were very close, and he graciously helped us finance our new-old house by obtaining the mortgage in his name and giving us a rent-to-own contract. He saw our vision.

Unfortunately, the neighborhood was horrible. We soon became accustomed to hearing gunshots and drunken neighbors screaming at one another. But inside the house was our little sanctuary, and I felt comfortable knowing there were four to six college boys living downstairs at any time for protection.

My life was so different now. I breathed a sigh of relief, as our payments were less than eight hundred dollars.

We got our routines down pat. Andréa and I mostly spent our days working on the house and our weekends camping or boating with what friends I had left or just our little family. I saw Zack only when he popped upstairs to say hello or get advice about some girl he was dating.

Andréa and I spent twenty-four hours a day together, and neither of us ever got tired of the other. We just had a really big love.

CHAPTER 4

Beautiful Chaos

March 4, 2012

THE NIGHT WE MET LIZ AND ERICA, ANDRÉA AND I went back to our hotel to spend time together. We dropped the surrogate subject and had a lovely date night.

However, I wasn't surprised when she wanted to talk about it first thing the next morning.

"Look, babe, I'm not going to tell you what to do. It's your decision," I told her as we lay in bed. "But we need to think hard about it. It's going to change our lives a lot."

"I could contribute toward the bills," she replied. "I don't like always relying on you."

"We don't need the money. I have plenty of money for the house." I got out of bed and pulled my sweats out of our overnight bag. "Let's go downstairs and talk about this at breakfast."

"My car is twelve years old. I could use a new one." Andréa was in bed naked, looking at the ceiling, still pondering how to sell this plan of hers to me. "Or we could take the kids on that trip to Disney World you keep talking about. *I* would love to do that for them. Me, not you—me! We could buy an old RV in Florida, like you've always wanted to, and drive it back home." She clearly wasn't about to give up.

"Come on, get dressed and we'll talk about it downstairs."

I already knew that I'd never tell Andréa what she could or couldn't do. We didn't work that way. If she felt she had to do this, of course I would support her. At the same time, I had to consider the stability and happiness of our family, not just Andréa's and my relationship. It had been only a year and a half. I didn't understand it, but she was clearly feeling an incredibly deep response to Liz and Erica's situation.

So at breakfast, I let her know the ball was in her court. Honestly, I was sure the whole idea was a phase that would pass.

Andréa decided she would email Erica the next day, but by the time we got home from our date night, Erica had already emailed her. After a few emails back and forth, we planned a dinner out with Liz and Erica. The plan was that we would meet with them again and see where things went.

I rather hoped they wouldn't go anywhere at all.

Liz and Erica Want This?

We didn't get together with them for several days. During that time, Andréa and I lay in bed every night talking about the surrogate idea and our upcoming meeting with the two women. This was always a time of peace and quiet in our house after the kids went to sleep.

"Liz and Erica have no idea what they're getting into," I laughed.

That first year with Jared and Julianna, I often wondered, *what the hell am I doing?* They're really cute, but they're not the kind of kids who can entertain themselves. The two seemed to be in constant competition to see who would be the center of attention, as if everyone around them was there strictly to fawn over them.

In the first few months before I left my job, I'd come home tired from work to find the kids running up and down the stairs screaming like banshees. Peace and quiet was a rarity. My new three thousand dollar TV (which Jared had nicked when he threw a Frisbee at it) would be blaring cartoons; meanwhile, Andréa would be typing away on her computer, searching for recipes for dinner, and completely oblivious to the madness. Some days I was tempted to turn around and run right back out the door and drive to the nearest bar.

The kids ate nonstop. Before dinner, they barked different orders at Andréa: "I want mac and cheese," Jared would clamor. "I want a peanut-butter-and-jelly sandwich," Julianna would yell with her charming little lisp. I'd watch in amazement as Andréa rushed around preparing the different requests. It wasn't long before I decided to intervene. I sat the kids down and firmly explained to them that their mother was not their slave or a short-order cook. And furthermore, they had to respect other people's things, and there would be no chaos anywhere in the house except in their own rooms. Of course, I was a fool to think they would listen and obey.

I loved them, but I was now leader of this group, and I definitely had to get the kids in line. I sternly put my foot down and established some guidelines. "My number-one rule is, the minute you're not thankful is the minute you lose that thing you're not thankful for," I told them. It took them a while to get it, but they quickly learned when trick-or-treating was cut short that first year. They had been so excited about all their candy, they were forgetting to say thank you.

In reality, growing up with me was particularly tough for four-year-old Jared. I had to remind him constantly, "Yes, you *are* very cute and wonderful—but the world does not revolve around you. You are not the center of everyone's universe, and your sister is just as important."

Jared was shocked. "She is not as important as me. I'm the boss, I'm special. Grandpa told me so," he said matter-of-factly, with an angelic smile on his face. Poor little Jared, he had to learn very quickly that that was not the case.

Even through the trials and tribulations of parenthood, I couldn't help but feel lucky. Andréa and I had an amazing love. Our life together was amazing too. It worked. She would tell me, "I love you more than anyone has ever loved anyone in the entire history of love." She joked that if she could exist on a deserted island with just me, that was where she would want to live, but her serious tone made me think she wasn't really joking. Sometimes I worried that she was too codependent on me. But I found that all four of us were growing closer, so maybe dependency wasn't an issue. Maybe it was just what it took for us to become a family.

Even though I was strict, I could be fun too, and I came into Jared and Julianna's lives early enough for them to see me as a parent. We'd walk around the house doing funny voices. Jared could even sing like Ethel Merman, which was a real hoot! Andréa was too shy to join in our shenanigans. But one time I heard her imitating a *South Park* song: "Do-do-do, do-do-do...sexual harassment...p-p-panda," and from then on I called her Panda.

But as corny as all that may sound, I do know people spend their whole lives wishing for the kind of deep, loving bond we have, and most never find it. Andréa and I always recognized what we had and were grateful for it. Even if we didn't have a lot of money, we had so much more. We wished everyone could find a family like ours, especially Liz and Erica.

"Maybe we could help fulfill this dream for them," Andréa said.

Running from the Monsters

In Andréa's eyes, I could do no wrong. She was still getting to know me. And then something happened that I couldn't help. Andréa would learn I had some not-so-wonderful traits.

We hadn't been together long, not quite a year. It was that first Halloween, my favorite holiday, even more so than Christmas. We were still establishing our roots as a family.

I started bringing down the Halloween decorations from the rafters in the garage: my life-size skeletons, huge spiders, and my favorite fifty-foot flying Grim Reaper. I hung him in the tree outside the front door so that he looked like he was coming straight out of the house. All the spooky characters were getting ready to make their appearances at my annual Halloween party!

How can I get the kids into the Halloween spirit? I thought. I really wanted them to love Halloween as much as I did. *What better way than to take them to the pumpkin patch!*

So my new little family and I got into my Ford Explorer, and off we went for our first autumn family tradition. The pumpkin patch off Highway 4 also had carnival rides. "This will be fun," I told the kids. "And you can each pick out your own pumpkin."

It was an unusually warm day for October, bright and sunny, but they were too excited for the cheery weather to dampen their spirits. "It feels like summer. It doesn't even feel like fall, darn it! I wish it were overcast and spooky," I grumbled a little, but I didn't really mean it. I'd been counting on this day to be the best ever, when I'd see the kids light up with great big smiles at all the Halloween decorations and rides.

As we drove into the parking lot, a big truck was unloading hundreds of fresh pumpkins.

"Look! We have a new batch to choose from," Andréa encouraged the kids. But they were already out of the car and running ahead of us through rows of pumpkins all neatly lined up. They were headed toward the entrance of the ride section.

Beyond the pumpkins was a vacant, rickety ticket booth. I signaled to a worker and asked him to come over and sell us ride tickets. We'd gotten there early, and the patch seemed pretty empty. "How cool, you guys! We have the place to ourselves!" I exclaimed, giving Jared and Julianna high fives. It was even better than I'd hoped for.

Only, as I looked around to help the kids choose their first ride, I saw that we weren't quite alone after all. There was a group of disabled people on a field trip with their care takers, emerging from a corner ride.

I had had two experiences with people like this. The first was when I was sentenced to community service at the home for disabled adults. The second was when I found my missing sister Rhonda—an occasion I didn't like to think of and had never told Andréa about. My heart sank. This was supposed to be our family-bonding day.

"Ah, man, do they have to be here today, of all days?" I said out loud to Andréa. She looked over at me with such a surprised expression that I wished I'd kept my mouth shut. But it was too late. I'd said it, and it was out. I tried to justify myself. "Now the kids are going to have to wait longer while they get those people out of their wheelchairs," I said angrily.

Andréa continued to look stunned.

"What?" I asked her. "Why are you staring at me?" I pretended I didn't know why she was shocked, though I knew how I must have sounded, and I started to spiral downhill, trying to justify my thoughts. "What if one of them has a leaky diaper or something, and poops on the ride? Do you think these people are going to clean it up?" I said, waving my hands. Andréa just stared at me without saying a word. "They're going to scare the kids. They're real-life monsters." I kept digging the hole deeper. "What if they want to hug Julianna and they start drooling on her?"

I tried to direct the kids to the ride farthest from the group. Of course, Jared and Julianna didn't want to go on it. They wanted to go on the ones the disabled kids were riding. I was defeated. "Maybe we should just come back," I told Andréa.

She patted my hand. "Well, let's eat lunch first then, okay?" she said.

Something inside me was screaming. All I wanted to do was get out of there, and I couldn't do it fast enough. I felt trapped, although I didn't want to look like a complete ass.

Andréa insisted we couldn't disappoint the kids, so I agreed we'd stay and eat our picnic. "Maybe they'll leave by the time we finish lunch," I told her. We sat on haystacks and pulled out the sandwiches Andréa had packed for us.

"Why can't we go on the rides?" Jared was upset.

"If you're going to complain, then we'll just leave," I barked at him. But I couldn't eat; I felt too sick to my stomach. A kid with Down syndrome came over to the haystacks and sat across from us as he opened his brown paper bag and pulled out his sandwich. I managed to smile politely at him, and rearranged the kids on their haystacks to look the other way. Andréa quietly ate her sandwich with her eyebrows raised at me and a puzzled look on her face.

When the kids were through eating, the group was still there. Andréa wouldn't let us leave until Jared and Julianna had gone on at least a few rides. So I led them to the bouncy house farthest from the disabled kids. By now they were just happy to be going on any ride. We left soon after, but I did let them select pumpkins on our way out.

As we were driving home, Andréa needed to get something off her chest. "Why do you have a phobia about disabled people?" she asked me. "Where does it come from?"

It was the first time I'd ever seen her look at me in a disappointed way. She seemed surprised that I was not perfect.

"I don't have a phobia about disabled people," I snapped as I stopped at a traffic light and looked over at her.

"Is it all disabled people you're afraid of?" she asked, her eyes wide in disbelief.

"No," I said sharply. Then I threw my hand in. "It's the ones who want to hug you and drool on you. They just kind of scare me, I guess." I thought for a moment. "Maybe it just hurts me to see people like that. I'd rather not be reminded."

That's when I told Andréa about my sister Rhonda.

What Happened to My Sister?

I had last seen Rhonda two years earlier, the year before Mom passed away.

Rhonda was well into her twenties by the time I was born, married and pregnant. When I was growing up, she was more like an aunt to me—an aunt I saw only once a year. She was the most beautiful of Mom's five kids—the spitting image of our mother. Beautiful as she was, Rhonda was plagued all her life with chronic illnesses. Mom thought she was an attention-seeking hypochondriac, and it put distance between them. Mom was never one to embrace complainers (neither am I), but there must have been something to Rhonda's illnesses. It is interesting that, like Mom, Rhonda ended up having not one but multiple brain aneurisms as a fairly young woman.

When Mom moved us to Texas for the sake of my brothers, who were getting into teenage trouble on the busy streets of southern California, we began to lose touch with Rhonda. Rhonda's occasional Christmas cards became no Christmas cards at all, and then Mom's cards came stamped "no longer at this address." We moved back to California eight years later. I didn't think much about it. I really didn't know her.

There were things I didn't understand about Mom, and Rhonda was one of them. Mom could have called Rhonda's ex-husband, whose phone number never changed and who was still close to Rhonda, to find out where she was. But for some reason, she never bothered. A few times Mom told me she thought Rhonda must have had another aneurysm and died. Maybe Mom didn't want to hear that news.

I eventually embraced my matriarch role and urged Mom to call to at least find out, but I didn't push it. Mom had her reasons, and I didn't want to step on her toes.

We did not hear from Rhonda again for more than ten years, but at last we finally did. Mom was in her eighties when she received a letter out of the blue. By this time, Mom weighed less than seventy-five pounds, and her days were numbered. According to the letter, Rhonda had in fact had a third aneurysm (or stroke), and this one had taken its toll. She was living in a rehabilitation center in southern California. After Mom read the letter, her relief went back to worry. She immediately wanted to know more. "I have a bad feeling about Rhonda, Kes," she told me. I was regional sales manager for my company at the time, and the job required me to travel frequently to southern California. Mom wanted me to visit Rhonda. "To make sure she's okay," she said. So, on my next business trip, I set aside a few hours to visit my sister. I found her son—my nephew Steven—on Facebook. Steven is only a year younger than I am, and we grew up with a cousin type of relationship until we left for Texas when

I was thirteen. He and I arranged a meeting to go see Rhonda at the rehabilitation center. I called Steven when I was on my way. He insisted on meeting me in the parking lot of the Shady Pines Center so that we could go in together. We agreed to meet at ten in the morning.

Me being me, I arrived twenty minutes early. The center was a one-story white building with nicely kept lawns attractively landscaped with exotic plantings. Feeling slightly reassured, I decided not to wait for Steven and went in.

I was in for a shock.

There were dazed patients sitting in wheelchairs. A man wearing a helmet was banging his head on the wall. *Is he retarded or something?* I wondered. There were confused people walking down the halls, mumbling to themselves.

What kind of rehabilitation hospital is this? It didn't seem like a hospital or any kind of treatment facility. *I must be in the wrong wing,* I thought.

A male employee came walking briskly by me. I stopped him and asked, "Can you tell me where Rhonda Thompson's room is?"

He smiled. "Go all the way down the hall and turn right. It's in the far corner of the hospital."

As I followed his directions through the long corridors, the walk seemed interminable. There was a weird smell everywhere—of baby powder and bleach. I was feeling more and more uneasy.

I finally got to the room in the corner. The door was already open, so I walked in. The room was larger and less formal than a typical hospital room. It had two sets of beds against the wall opposite from each other. There were three patients in the room and one empty madeup bed. Two patients were elderly ladies who looked asleep in their beds on one side of the room, and a third was a bald, obese woman sitting in a chair in the corner on the other side. She was clutching a can of Pepsi with deformed hands and drooling all over herself as she tried unsuccessfully to take a drink.

Where is my sister? Puzzled and repelled, I walked out of the room to look for a nurse while holding my stomach, which was now very queasy.

"Can you tell me how to find a patient named Rhonda Thompson?" I asked a nurse in the corridor. She walked me back to that same room.

"She's here," the nurse told me, smiling and waving her hand at the door I had just come out of. I wanted to yell at her, *No, my sister's not in there.* I didn't want to go back into that room.

But I had to prove that I'd already looked. Humoring the woman, I searched the room again for Rhonda. I glanced quickly past the obese woman with clawed hands. And then my eyes came back to her. Suddenly I realized: This woman was my sister Rhonda.

She was unrecognizable.

This can't be my beautiful sister! What am I going to tell Mom? I was shocked and disgusted. The room started to whirl, and I felt like throwing up.

I almost turned and ran out. But the woman with clawed hands spoke to me. "Kessy?" she quavered in a guttural, barely intelligible voice.

I knew I had to turn around and face her, so I did. Still fighting every desire to turn and run, instead I walked over and sat down in a chair that the nurse brought in for me. I sat next to my sister, smiled, and nodded as we started to make small talk. I was graceful on the outside—after all, I was my mother's daughter—but inside I felt disgust and despair.

We ended up having some sort of conversation. Some of the time, I felt like she was making sense. She seemed to be "in there," especially when she asked about our mother, but mostly, I didn't have a clue about what she was saying. It was awful. I couldn't look away or she would know what I was thinking. I certainly did not want to hurt her feelings, in case she knew what was really going on. I stared at the oldest of Mom's five children. The luckiest one of us, once graced with stunning good looks, was now twisted into a grotesque, drooling shell of a woman, her tongue protruding as she blathered on without making sense.

Steven finally arrived and was not happy with me. "You stinker," he said with an irritated tone, but he did manage to smile at me. I hadn't seen Steven since he was twelve. Now a man, he stood tall, handsome,

and all grown-up. Unfortunately, I could not celebrate the moment. I now knew why he had wanted to meet me in the parking lot. He must have written the letter to Mom. My sister might have dictated it to some degree, but there was no way she could have written it.

Rhonda had pooped in her pants, and Steven and I waited behind a curtain in the vacant corner of the room as an orderly changed her diaper. I just looked at him. It was awkward. We didn't know what to say to each other. Once Rhonda was cleaned up, the orderly wheeled her outside so she could enjoy the sun as Steven and I followed behind.

I did not know Rhonda very well, but as we walked down the hall, I remembered how much she had loved to sunbathe. We sat outside on a bench while Rhonda, still in her wheelchair, held her chin up high to enjoy the warmth of the sun on her face and Steven and I exchanged small talk.

As we chatted about other family members, Rhonda listened intently. I exchanged looks with Steven, as if he could read my thoughts from my expression. *Why didn't you tell me about Rhonda's condition when we talked on the phone?*

After half an hour, I decided to make an excuse that I had to get to work. I was literally sick to my stomach and knew I needed to get out of there fast. I left Rhonda and Steven in front of the building, Rhonda still enjoying the sunshine. I got into my Ford Explorer, backed out of the parking space, and waved to them as I drove off. As soon as I was around the corner and far enough away, I pulled into a McDonald's parking lot, got out of the car, leaned my arms over the hood, and threw up, while crying almost hysterically.

I knew my sister had no idea of my disgust; I could play parts beautifully, but seeing Rhonda in that condition was like being back in that horrible home for disabled adults. I felt the same kind of sickness, shock, disgust, and fear. But this was worse, because Rhonda was my sister. What kind of sister was I to be feeling this way about her? But I did, and I couldn't help it.

I called Mom and told her the truth. I hated to; she was eighty-two and weak. But Mom still had all her faculties, and she would never have

wanted me to lie to her, even if the truth caused her pain. She always faced the things she had to. At least she now knew where Rhonda had been all these years.

I told Andréa about my sister, but I still couldn't bring myself to speak about my time at the disabled facility, a haunting secret that I kept trying to ignore. I should have known better, because after I told Andréa about Rhonda, she still loved me and kept me on a pedestal just the same. That was Andréa. She continued to love me, maybe even more, warts and all.

And then I locked that horrible day away, back into its deep crevice in my memory, hoping to never be reminded of it again.

Life was great after all!

CHAPTER 5

We Can Be Heroes

ANDRÉA WAS SERIOUS ABOUT THE SURROGATE THING. As we talked it over, I could see that she felt in her heart of hearts that this was a "good" thing to do. She wanted to make Liz and Erica's dreams come true. Even though she kept trying to sell it to me as her doing her part for the family financially, I knew there had to be more to it. Andréa was not one to care about money, and we had enough, and only a few bills. We lived simply, within our means, so I knew money was not her motivation. I felt like Andréa harbored a lot of guilt—I thought maybe over not being the perfect daughter, letting her parents down, and then marrying a drunk ex-con and not making something meaningful out of her life. I knew she felt this was her moment to make a difference.

"Babe, I'm not sure why you're doing this, but I'll always support you," I assured her. I agreed to move forward with the surrogacy and share my beautiful Andréa with Liz and Erica for the next ten or eleven months.

I did agree with Erica's original offer to compensate Andréa for the inconvenience, pain, and suffering. After all, it would be a year out of Andréa's and my life, and the surrogacy would require us to make some sacrifices. We decided to postpone our small beach wedding, and we gave up any ideas about going on vacation or doing any fun sports. This was going to be taxing on her body; it was a lot for her to do for them.

But what did surrogates actually make?

We spent an evening researching online. We ended up opening up a confusing can of worms, as the compensation seemed to range anywhere from ten to forty thousand dollars. It depended greatly on whether Andréa was using her own egg (which we were), using Liz and Erica's, or using a donor's. Honestly, we really didn't know where to start or what to expect, so we split the difference and wrote up a proposal for Erica and Liz. We also found out that since they were going to use Andréa's eggs, they would be required to adopt the baby once it was born.

Andréa started making plans to include Liz and Erica in every aspect of the pregnancy. She was starting to become over-the-moon excited for them. Getting pregnant and making their dreams come true was all we talked about. There was never a question in Andréa's mind what wonderful parents they would be.

"I want to give them the full mommy experience," she told me one night, her eyes shining as she started making plans while we lay in bed. She was staring at the ceiling as she talked to me, but she was really thinking out loud and talking to herself. She went on and on. She wanted them to make an audiotape to talk to their baby in utero so he or she would know their voices. She wanted them as involved as if they themselves were the ones who were pregnant: "Kind of like husbands, you know?" she explained. "The parent, just not the one carrying the child." It meant the world to Andréa to make this baby for them.

She and I were a team. It didn't take long before I started to become as committed to this as she was. Admittedly, seeing my very beautiful Andréa pregnant was a sweet thought. I couldn't wait.

The morning after Andréa daydreamed about handing over a beautiful baby to Liz and Erica, I was getting ready in the bathroom for my day, thinking about what we were about to do. I could feel a presence outside the bathroom door. I opened it and there was Mom.

"Why in the hell would you have a baby for someone else?" she said with concern. *"If they can't have a baby, then they can't have a baby. That's that."* Mom shrugged her shoulders nonchalantly.

I laughed as I was brushing my teeth. *"It's important to Andréa, Ma. It's an unselfish thing she's doing,"* I said out loud just as I was starting to rinse. Realizing that I might not be alone, I looked out the bathroom door to see whether Andréa or the kids might hear me and think I was crazy. Luckily, they were downstairs.

"You don't even know these women."

"You're right about that, Ma," I said. I put the toothbrush back into its holder and pondered what she'd said. *"You are right. We really don't know them very well,"* I agreed, and nodded thankfully to Mom's apparition. *"And we need to change that."*

I walked out of the bathroom and found Andréa eating cereal at the dining room table. "We need to get to know them first, Andréa," I told her. I didn't need to tell her whom I was talking about.

She looked up. "Uh, okay."

She agreed with Mom too.

Agreeing to Agree
March 9, 2012

After a few emails and texts back and forth, we decided to meet Liz and Erica for dinner. Erica chose a little Italian restaurant called Forno Vecchio, midway between where we lived in Antioch and where they lived in San Jose.

Andréa and I arrived early, as we usually do. It was still light outside, and it didn't feel quite like dinnertime yet. The restaurant was in a quaint uptown strip of stores and eateries. We walked in and were greeted by a young hostess in black pants and a white button-down shirt. After she told us we could sit where we wanted, we chose a table for four against the mirrored wall to give us privacy. We sat together on the wall side so we could look outward and face Liz and Erica when they arrived. Underneath, we were very anxious, and it felt good to be sitting side by side. We were in this together, however things turned out. We each ordered a glass of wine to ease our nerves.

Andréa and I had set a goal for the evening: We wanted to get an idea of who Erica and Liz were and what kind of parents they would be. Would they provide Andréa's biological child with a good life? Would they love this baby? Most important, we wanted an informal agreement that we'd occasionally be able to see the baby, as "aunties."

It wasn't long at all before Liz and Erica walked through the door. They were both very chic, as if they'd just come from high-pressure management jobs in Silicon Valley. We got up to greet and hug them. As we sat back down, our waiter came to light the candle and asked Liz and Erica what they would like to drink. Like us, they ordered wine.

For the first few minutes, we all made uncomfortable and shallow small talk, which I find incredibly annoying and meaningless. It was a relief when the waiter came and we ordered.

Every detail of that evening has remained vividly in my memory, even down to what we ate. Andréa ordered vegetarian lasagna, while I had meat lasagna. Liz ordered risotto, and Erica wanted a salad. Luckily, at that point, the wine kicked in, and I was able to switch gears from the small talk to the reason we were all there.

"So, why do you want a baby so badly?" I asked them bluntly.

As Erica took the lead, it felt like we were on a first date with a suitor who was really attracted to us. Part of me felt as if we were receiving a sales pitch. Erica talked about how much they loved each other and had always wanted kids. "It's been my dream," she said. "We make a lot of money and could afford to give the baby a very good life."

I listened to her with all my senses on alert.

Liz sure doesn't talk much. I wonder if this is their dream or just Erica's.

I needed to know that they were both committed, and I needed to protect Andréa. "Whose dream is this?" I asked.

Liz quickly chimed in, as if she were reading my mind: "We both want this."

Erica nodded in agreement. "Yes. We both want this."

Liz told us that she had actually wanted the baby so badly that after Erica failed to get pregnant, she herself started fertility treatments. She had even participated in a study at Stanford in hopes that they could get pregnant. "Nothing worked, and it only stressed me out more," Liz confided. She spoke with confidence, even though she was less animated than Erica.

The more they told us, the worse Andréa and I felt for them. Their longing for a child was so real, and they had suffered so much. No wonder Liz seemed withdrawn. Andréa was close to tears beside me. We communicated wordlessly with each other, and then suddenly the words came out: I told them we would surrogate for them. It felt right, the only thing to do.

"Can we see the child as aunties from time to time as he or she grows up?" I requested. Fearful that I'd put them off, I explained. "The thought of Andréa having a child somewhere out in the universe whom we don't know and never see doesn't feel warm and fuzzy to me. I have to watch out for her." I gave an uneasy smile.

Andréa pinched my hand under the table and gave me a shut-up look as she spoke. "We don't expect contact, though maybe you can send us pictures once a year?" she suggested.

I looked at Andréa and was just about to disagree with her, but Erica put her hand up and stopped me midsentence.

"We fully expect for you to be able to see the baby from time to time." Liz and Erica had obviously already given this thought. "We'd invite you to family functions, birthday parties, and important things like that."

Andréa chimed in as if doing damage control, "The baby never has to know who I am."

But Erica reassured us and informed us of their plan: Once the child was old enough, they would be honest and tell him or her, "Your aunt Andréa is your biological mother. She helped us have you." Erica spoke as if she were already talking to the child.

She made me feel better. I wasn't completely sure that Liz was onboard, though, because she was so quiet.

I looked at Andréa and spoke plainly: "Someday, Andréa, we will have an eighteen-year-old knocking on our door wanting to know who you are." I wanted to be perfectly sure Liz and Erica understood that I wasn't keen on zero contact and expected them to keep their agreement. Erica reiterated that they had planned all along to be honest and open as the child grew up, and that we'd certainly see the baby.

As much as Andréa hated it, we spent the rest of the evening talking about what Andréa would be going through, the risks, and the compensation, which we agreed would be in the middle of the extreme discrepancies in averages paid to surrogates.

Finally, everything was arranged. We would do this. Andréa would get pregnant using donor sperm and her own egg. Liz wanted to use a Middle-Eastern donor so the baby would look more like her. Once the baby was born, she and Erica would have to adopt it from Andréa and me.

At the end of dinner, I pulled out my wallet. Erica put her hand on mine and said, "We have this. It's the least we can do." We thanked them, said goodnight, and went our separate ways.

Andréa and I talked it over on our drive home. We both felt good about them, but for some reason I couldn't quite identify, I continued to have misgivings. "We still really don't know these women. We know what they're saying, but we don't know *them*."

Andréa was sure, though. "They want this baby so badly, Keston. They'll love it. And they can clearly provide for it." She felt even more confident that she wanted to do this than before. Her doubts, if she had ever had any, were gone. Her heart was sure.

They had told us during dinner that while Erica made six figures, Liz made double or almost triple her salary. They were both successful in their professional lives in the Silicon Valley tech world.

"The baby would have a nice life, Keston," Andréa said as I drove us back through the now-dark valley heading home.

I couldn't argue with that.

Anyone who would go through so much to have a child surely deserves to be a parent, I thought. I pushed back my reservations and listened to

Andréa's heart, which wasn't hard after hearing all Liz and Erica had been through. I was firmly on board.

Now we were going to have to tell Andréa's family, and explain this to Jared and Julianna. What in the world would they say?

Congratulations, You Are Not Going to Be Grandparents!

We knew this would be confusing for four-year-old Julianna and seven-year-old Jared.

At our family dinner the next night, between bites of the stuffed chicken and orzo Andréa had prepared so masterfully, I announced to the kids, "Mama is going to make a baby for some friends." Andréa was quiet.

Julianna giggled, while Jared looked puzzled. "How is she going to do that?" he asked.

We weren't counting on such directness. Andréa and I were fumbling through awkward explanations when Jared hit us with another direct question: "Will the baby be our brother or sister?"

"No, the baby will not belong to us," I answered.

Jared went on eating for a moment, and then said, "Okay."

Julianna just listened, still smiling and being silly. And that was that!

Next we had to tackle Andréa's parents. That wasn't quite so easy. They had divorced when she was twelve, and it had affected her terribly. She had become a hellion teen.

Her relationship with her mother was strained at best. As a preteen, Andréa tried to punish both of her parents (as well as their new spouses) with her bad attitude and reckless behavior. Her taking the responsibility and blame as a teen vixen for seducing their well-respected adult family friend, only to go on to marry and get pregnant by an alcoholic ex-con, certainly didn't help.

In her past, she'd constantly made bad decisions, which she regretted. She was desperate for their love and approval. *Would they think this was another bad decision?*

Andréa told her mother first.

The kids lovingly called their grandmother and favorite grandparent Tutu. "It means 'grandmother' in Hawaiian. Tutu's mother spent time growing up in the islands," Andréa enlightened me.

Tutu was very private, a shy yet classy lady. Half Korean and half American, she was pretty, poised, graceful, quiet, reserved, and a very involved, caring grandparent to Jared and Julianna. She enjoyed the finer things in life and showed her love with gifts. Andréa thought it was because her mother had grown up with so little herself. Andréa was a blond version of her mother, with the same beautiful almond shaped eyes and tall, slender body.

Andréa had mixed feelings about her mother. "My mom can be cold and unemotional," she would tell me. It still hurt and baffled her at times. "Even though she doesn't say she's disappointed in me, she makes me feel like she is," was the way she put it. Yet when it came to her grandchildren, she bought the kids material things, just as she'd done when Andréa was little, but she also did more. Tutu was downright silly. She'd get down on their level and play games with them. That was what the kids really loved about her. As close as she was to Jared and Julianna, how was she going to react to this baby who would not be a grandchild?

I could tell that Andréa yearned for a more meaningful relationship with her mother. It was sad. She would tell me that she could never please her mother. She gave up trying, but I could see beyond her façade, and I could tell she wanted more than anything to be close to her mother. It broke my heart.

"Panda," I told her, "that goes two ways. You're an adult now. Your mom is shy. Maybe she's not sure how to talk to you. I don't hear you trying to sit down and talk to her."

"I've always been a failure to her," Andréa responded sadly. "She doesn't talk to me, Keston, not real talk. It's always just small talk." Andréa started to speak faster, as if she wanted the conversation to be over, but needed to get something off her chest. "I always remembered wanting to hug my mom when I was little, and she always pushed me away. I guess I smothered her. But she tells my kids how much she loves them, hugs them, and still today she never tells me she loves me. I always say it, but only when I hang up the phone." There it was. With a twinge of jealousy at the love her children received from Tutu, Andréa had blurted out the truth.

There was reason for her pain. Not only were Jared and Julianna the apples of Tutu's eye, but they in return thought she hung the moon. No wonder Andréa had mixed emotions about her mother's close relationship with the children.

Andréa told her mother in an email about our decision to surrogate. Needless to say, Tutu did not react positively.

I was putting up drywall in the basement when Andréa came down to tell me about her mother's response. "It's just as I expected. She isn't happy with me surrogating. She thinks it's awful, and says how weird it will be to have a grandchild out there whom she'll never know."

"Did you tell her we'll be seeing the baby as aunties, and that the baby will be attending family functions?" I asked.

"No," she said, shrugging as if to say there was no point. She couldn't talk about it anymore.

Either way, it was one down, one to go.

Andréa wasn't worried about telling her father. Boppi was sixty-three years young, and very Swiss. When I first met him, Boppi's accent was so thick, I couldn't understand a word he said. I had to look to Andréa for interpretation, even though he was speaking English. He'd come to America in the seventies from a small town in Switzerland, and was a very European, open-minded, and loving man. Andréa felt close to him. When I first met her, she used to tell me, "My dad is just a great man, Keston. Everyone respects him."

"Why?" I asked.

"He's never judgmental, and he always listens," she told me proudly. "I know if I need anything, he'll always be there for me."

Like Tutu, Boppi was also an amazing grandparent. Jared and Julianna called him "Grossboppi," which is Swiss for "grandfather." He filled the father-figure role in their lives and spent quality time with both kids. Boppi was the kind of man who would happily spend eight hours at the park playing with them, or take them hiking through town or the nearby hills. He was firm and didn't spoil them, but he took the time to talk to them, and, more important, he listened.

Andréa had told me about Boppi, "Actions speak louder than words, and while my dad isn't great about saying he loves me, his actions show me every day how much he does."

The way I had Mom, Andréa had Boppi. He was the first person she went to for advice. "I might hear a short lecture, but he accepts my decisions and is always a hundred percent supportive of me," she told me.

Boppi's partner Robin was more of a challenge for Andréa. Their relationship was somewhat strained. A no-nonsense, blunt lady (a lot like me), Robin could be mean-spirited in her delivery. Even shorter than I, Robin barely stood five feet tall in heels. She was a very dark-skinned African-American, and the saying about dynamite coming in small packages described her perfectly. Early on, I got the impression that Robin was annoyed by and not sympathetic to Andréa's life choices. Andréa and I agreed that she might have been jealous of Andréa's relationship with Boppi.

Andréa was much more nonchalant about telling Boppi that we had decided to do the surrogate thing. She didn't push it. She was all right with waiting until her thirtieth birthday party, just a week away.

After Andréa told me about Tutu's reaction, I figured both her parents would be more accepting if they met Liz and Erica. Even though Boppi already knew Erica, he had not seen her in many years.

Consequently, I added the two women to the party invitation, but also privately texted Erica. "Hey, girl, I think it would be good for Andréa's folks to meet you and Liz. It's important, so can you guys come to Andréa's thirtieth birthday party?"

"Absolutely," Erica texted back within seconds.

"Great! We'll see you Saturday," I typed. I was very happy with myself. I thought for sure they would impress Tutu and Boppi and put their minds at ease. Also, Andréa and I could get to know them a little better.

The following Saturday morning Andréa and I were up early getting ready for her big day. Since it was Saint Patrick's Day, Andréa was busy preparing a corned-beef-and-cabbage feast. She was chopping onions, mixing sauces, and brining the beef. I picked up the Guinness, Bailey's, and Jameson for Irish Car Bombs, and then spent the afternoon setting up microphones for my band that was briefly reuniting, while the kids tried to help clean the house. The day went by quickly, and in what seemed like no time at all, guests were starting to arrive.

We had at least fifty family members and friends, many of the latter lesbians. I'd decorated the house to the hilt. On anything and everything, I hung either "Happy Thirtieth" decorations or St. Patrick's Day four-leaf clovers. The whole house was filled with the mouthwatering aroma of Andréa's cooking.

As the house began to fill up, we sent the kids to bed. We wished Liz and Erica could have come earlier to meet them, but it was adult time now.

My band had just finished playing "Whole Lotta Love" when I saw Liz and Erica coming through the front door. Excited, I switched the PA over to recorded music and grabbed Andréa, who was downing an Irish Car Bomb at the bar with a bunch of friends. We went over to greet Liz and Erica.

We both hugged them, and then turned around to introduce them to Tutu, who was standing close by, and Andréa's stepfather Scott, as well as Andréa's aunt, Tutu's sister Sharon. We filled Sharon in on our plans soon after the introductions. Luckily, Sharon was much more outgoing than Tutu. She broke the ice immediately with stories about her own trials with infertility, and the group began chatting.

As Andréa and I were pulled away to greet new guests, I heard Sharon tell Liz and Erica, "How lucky you are to have Andréa doing this for you."

Tutu was not getting involved in the conversation, but she did stand there with her arms crossed and listened. I couldn't tell whether it was just shyness or disapproval.

Fate will have to take its course!

As the party went on late into the evening, I saw that Boppi was talking with Erica.

Oh, no, we haven't said anything to him! I'd better get Andréa before Erica says anything. I nervously hoped they were talking about family, since Boppi knew Erica as Kris's ex.

I quickly found Andréa, who was having fun and was confused as to why I was pulling her away, and hustled her over to them. "Hey Boppi," I interrupted, "Andréa is thinking about surrogating for Liz and Erica."

There was a long pause as he looked at me without saying a word. Andréa stood there unable to speak, waiting for his reaction. I gave him a brief history of how we had come to that decision. He just nodded without making any comment. At that point, Andréa and I were reluctantly dragged away to entertain other guests.

After many birthday shots, a lot of delicious food, and a great deal of fun, people started leaving. Liz and Erica had a long drive home, so they also left. There was finally time for me to give Andréa a big birthday kiss. We were saying goodbye to people and noticed Boppi sitting alone on the stairs. Andréa, who doesn't usually drink much, was glassy-eyed and full of smiles as we walked up to him hand in hand.

After standing next to him for a moment, I realized Andréa wasn't going to talk. She might have had one shot too many.

"So, what do you think?" I asked him, not wanting to beat around the bush.

"It's a very big thing to do," he replied in his thick Swiss accent. Then he added, looking directly at Andréa, "It's very nice of you." As always, Boppi was supportive of his daughter, whatever she did. He told us he believed Andréa was capable of giving up her biological child, and he had no problem with it. Other than that, he never volunteered another word.

The party was over, everyone in our family knew of our plans, and we were moving ahead.

Is There a Gyno in the House?
March 19, 2012

We had our plan and everyone was on board. We knew what we were going to do. But first we had to get rid of one little problem: We had to get Andréa's hormone-releasing IUD removed.

Andréa had had it "installed" years ago so she wouldn't have to deal with the hassles of menstruation and hadn't had a period in many years.

That Monday morning after her birthday, Andréa was upstairs in bed when she called her regular doctor to ask him for a referral to a gynecologist. He always seemed to ask odd and inappropriate questions, and we had never been comfortable with him.

I came upstairs just as she was hanging up. She looked upset. "He won't give me a referral. He wants to see me himself."

To top it off, we would have to wait a month for an appointment.

I was furious. "Are you kidding me? I'm going to call him back. He needs to give you an ob-gyn referral now!"

"No, don't piss him off. I don't want to make waves." She looked at me and gave a big sigh.

"Panda, that idiot needs to know that every woman has a right to choose who looks up her fucking vagina."

To my surprise, Andréa looked shocked.

"I wish you wouldn't say that word," she blurted out.

"What word?" I asked, bewildered. She didn't say anything; she just looked shy and shaked her head. Then I got it. "You mean *vagina?*"

"Yes," she nodded.

"Uh, every woman has a vagina, Andréa." I couldn't believe Andréa, a grown woman, was uncomfortable with the word.

She thought about it for a few seconds and then tried to explain.

"I know, it's just that that word is kind of…"

"Vulgar?" I filled in the blank. I was trying to bite my tongue.

"Yes."

You have to be kidding me! I gave her a long, puzzled stare, shocked at her innocence.

I finally responded in the most cheerful, patient manner I could muster, "Well, can I use the word *va-jay-jay* then? I mean, that should be okay. It's what we call it to Julianna, right?"

"Yes, that sounds better." She seemed relieved and then gave me a crooked smile. "Anyway, I think we can do this without the doctor."

I should have known that Andréa would have an alternative plan. She was always ingenious that way.

"I was reading that many women remove IUDs by themselves," she said.

"Uh-huh…and how do they do that?"

"You can actually feel the strings and pull it out yourself."

"You've gotta be kidding!" I tried to picture how a woman could do that.

"No, seriously, they say it's as easy as removing a tampon," she told me with confidence and a wicked smile, like the cat who swallowed the canary.

Why do I have the feeling that she's trying to talk me into something?

"Keston, go online and look it up. They say it's easy, and I can feel the strings with my fingers. We just have to pull them."

To humor her, I climbed into the bed beside her and we began looking up IUD removal on my laptop. And just as Andréa had described, there were many forums and chats with women who had removed their own IUDs. The consensus seemed to be that you could do it if you could feel the strings, if you could actually grab them.

"If you think you can pull it out, you should try," I told her. Again, I should have known that Andréa was a step ahead of me.

"Well, I can feel them, but I can't grab them from this angle."

Darn, that's too bad, I thought, shaking my head.

After a few seconds of trying to puzzle out how she could rearrange the angle, I glanced over and saw that she had a devious smile on her face, and I realized exactly what Andréa was trying to sell me.

"No way," I told her bluntly, waving my hand back and forth

emphatically. "No, I am not doing it. I am not sticking my fingers that deep…I would have to practically put my *entire* hand up in your vagi… va-jay-jay."

Andréa sat looking at me silently as if she were about to cry.

Darn it!

Within a few minutes, I found myself between Andréa's legs in a very clinical, unsexy, and much different position than I ever thought I would be, fishing for those elusive IUD strings.

"This is so weird," I told her, and I couldn't help but laugh as I saw more of Andréa's va-jay-jay than I could have ever imagined. I looked up to make sure the curtains were tightly closed. "Can you imagine what our neighbors would think if they got a shot of this?" I started spewing out lesbian jokes: "What's the difference between a bowling ball and a lesbian?" I giggled as I tried to find and pinch the strings between my fingers, only for them to slip away as soon as I found them. "You can only get three fingers in a bowling ball!"

"Be serious, Keston!" Andréa scolded me, but I couldn't be, and soon she was laughing too.

Unfortunately, my fingers were too short. I thought I'd found the strings a few times, but I could barely reach them. "They're too slippery!" I told Andréa. "Maybe I could do it if I could see them." Suddenly I had an idea, and I ran downstairs to grab a pair of thin salad tongs. A few minutes later, I was back upstairs and in my amateur gynecologist position, this time with a handy tool that I had boiled in water. "If I could open the tongs up just a little in there, I might be able to see the strings," I explained to Andréa, who was looking at me doubtfully.

"Well, give it a try," she managed to say.

A few seconds later I pronounced, "They work! I can see the strings!" But now I realized I couldn't get my fingers around the tongs to grab them. I had another brilliant idea: "Maybe I can grab the slippery little suckers better with the tongs," I said, in deep concentration. I got a good look at where the strings were, and then moved the tongs in deeper. Maneuvering them around the strings, I closed them tightly, not at all sure I even had the strings in their grip. "Okay, here goes!" I warned Andréa. Very slowly, I pulled the tongs out, expecting them to be empty. But there on the end was a little plastic T and the two infamous strings. "I did it!" I yelled in triumph.

It really was as easy and painless as pulling out a tampon.

Andréa was elated! I was her hero. We burst out laughing and hugging each other. Andréa finally pulled herself together. "Okay, babe, I'm ready to text Erica."

So much for doctor weird dude. We were good to go!

CHAPTER 6

The Journey Begins

April 22, 2012

LIZ AND ERICA EMAILED THE FINAL AGREEMENT THAT they had their lawyer draft for us to look over. It felt strange to be so businesslike over such a human matter, but we knew it had to be that way. Andréa and I looked over the document together, and we thought it was pretty straightforward.

The agreement spelled everything out: We would use Andréa's eggs and donor sperm of Liz and Erica's choice. We would use Liz and Erica's fertility doctor. Once pregnant, Andréa would be compensated for her "pain and suffering," to be spread out in monthly payments during the pregnancy due on the first of each month. She would also receive a retainer fee upfront. Once the baby was born, because it would be Andréa's biological child, and since she and I were partners, we agreed to let Liz and Erica adopt it. Also, Andréa and I would be reimbursed for our travel expenses, and if Andréa had to take fertility drugs in the form of injections, Liz and Erica would compensate her for further pain and suffering. There would be additional compensation if Andréa were to become pregnant with twins. Andréa would have the right to choose reduction if there were more than two fetuses (meaning she had the right to abort any fetuses beyond two). However, Liz and Erica could choose to terminate the pregnancy for medical reasons, but if they made that choice after twenty weeks of gestation, they would have to compensate Andréa in full. Liz and Erica agreed to obtain life insurance for Andréa, with Jared and Julianna listed as beneficiaries. Both Andréa and I were required to sign the agreement.

I told Andréa that we needed to get the surrogacy agreement signed and finalized "before you do anything else." At the time, I had no idea what we were about to embark upon.

"Look, I know you don't like to talk business and money, but still—" I was saying when Andréa stopped me.

"I know, I know," she said. "I'll text them and let them know we need to meet and sign the agreement before I do any inseminations," she assured me.

Liz and Erica were eager to get started. "The sooner the better," Erica texted. "We aren't getting any younger."

We decided to meet them again for dinner, this time to sign the agreement and officially kick off the baby-making adventure.

Andréa and I took Jared and Julianna with us, so we needed to choose a kid-friendly place. This was to be the first time Liz and Erica would meet the kids. I couldn't help but be excited for them to see what their future child might look like. Both Jared and Julianna were beautiful kids. Jared, with his long eyelashes, blue eyes, blond hair, fair skin, and perfect lips, looked like a little-boy version of his mother. He was very book-smart, but he tended to be gullible too. Julianna could really get at him, and she was clearly the leader of the two, even though she was two-and-a-half years younger. She looked like a true "California girl." Her blond hair, which she insisted on having high-lighted with bright pink streaks, accented her tan skin and blue-green eyes. Julianna was a lot like me: She could easily command a room. She was also a mischief-maker, often talking Jared into making bad decisions. These two could win over the hardest of hearts!

Because I was a strict mom, they both knew they were expected to be well mannered. It was very important to me that they be "thank you" and "yes, please" kinds of kids. We knew Liz and Erica would go home and talk about them.

"What's better than pizza?" Erica suggested. So we agreed to meet at the Gay Nineties Pizza Company in Pleasanton.

It was a funky little corner restaurant in the old part of town. The interior was an odd L-shaped room. Everything was wood: a long wood bar, wood tables, and wood booths with red-and-white-checked tablecloths. There were old license plates and antique car parts on the walls.

Andréa, the kids, and I arrived early and picked out a table big enough for all of us, smack in the middle of the narrow dining room. Soon Liz and Erica arrived with Erica's niece Brittany in tow. Brittany was living with them while going to college in the Bay Area. She had long brown hair and looked like a sweet girl.

"This place is known for making the best pizza in Pleasanton!" Erica told us as they sat down. We ordered two large pizzas and salad. Jared and Julianna used their best manners and were being their usual darling selves, coloring on their paper menus with Brittany's help.

This meeting was the first time we noticed how awkward Liz seemed around children, though. She tried to talk to them, but I don't think she knew what to say or how to get down to their level. It seemed like she was forcing herself to talk to them. Erica, on the other hand, was a natural. She went to the kids' end of the table and told Jared and Julianna, who were busy coloring, "I like to color too," and she sat down and started talking to them about their artwork. Liz stayed with us at the other end while she watched in amazement as Erica conversed with Jared and Julianna. She had a funny look on her face, as if she thought the kids were from another planet.

Before we knew it, the pizzas and salad had come and we began eating. It wasn't until we'd finished and wiped the tomato sauce off Jared's and Julianna's faces that we finally focused on the business at hand. Liz brought out two copies of the contracts they had both already signed. Andréa and I signed both copies and kept one copy for ourselves. Then Liz presented Andréa with a big surprise: She handed her a check for the retainer.

Andréa was startled.

"Oh, you don't have to give this to me until your doctor has checked me out," she told Liz.

"No, go ahead and take it now," Liz insisted as Erica nodded in agreement.

"Well, I won't cash it until your doctor gives us the green light," Andréa stated firmly. She didn't feel comfortable taking the check. She held on to it for weeks before finally depositing it into her bank account.

We now had begun the journey of trying to get Andréa pregnant. "It will take one, maybe two tries," Andréa estimated, and I agreed.

As we were about to leave, I brought out my wallet. We certainly didn't expect Liz and Erica to pay, but Erica again said, "Put that away, we have this," as she handed her credit card to the waitress.

"Hey, you guys don't need to pay every time we meet. We'd like to be friends and not have you think we have expectations like that," I insisted to Liz and Erica. But they had already paid, so all we could do was thank them. Then we said our goodnights and left.

On our way home, the kids settled down in the back and fell asleep, while Andréa and I talked about the meeting, particularly Liz's awkwardness with small children. "That was amusing—and eye-opening," Andréa remarked.

I laughed and agreed. "Well, Liz will have to get past that."

"Their dynamic is interesting. Erica is going to be the fun-loving mom, while Liz will be the tough don't-break-the-rules mom," I said, and added, "But when their child earns her respect, it will be very valuable to them both."

The next day Erica texted Andréa; she had already set up an appointment with their fertility doctor, Dr. Santos.

And We're Off
May 9, 2012

Dr. Santos's office in Los Gatos was an eighty-mile drive from our house in Antioch. As my GPS (whom I call "Carmen") led us on the journey. Andréa read our horoscopes out loud for entertainment as I drove. That morning, we found the horoscopes to be very entertaining indeed. Andréa's read that she was in a position to be a "giver of life."

Coincidence? We wondered.

We met outside Dr. Santos's office, which was in one of those typical medical strips in the heart of a residential area. We were all excited as we said hello to one another at the fountain right outside the office door. We went in together and Liz checked us in. The waiting room was small, but at least it had nice high-backed leather couches that gave you the feeling it was an upscale place. Liz came back with paperwork for Andréa to fill out. As soon as she was finished answering the medical questionnaire, a nurse opened the door to the examination rooms, and we were called in. The nurse, Liz, and Erica greeted one another like old friends. She led us down a short hall into an exam room.

The room was very small; there wasn't much room left around the examining table, a rolling doctor's chair, and a small sink. On the light cream walls were corkboards with hundreds of pictures of the doctor holding newborn babies.

I had to squeeze into the corner at Andréa's head while she lay on the examining table. The nurse who'd brought us back told Andréa to undress from the waist down and then left the room. Andréa looked horrified. *In front of everyone?* How could she find any privacy in this tiny area? Eventually, she managed it behind a closed curtain, with Liz and Erica waiting together on the other side by the door. We talked nervously through the curtain until Andréa gave them the okay to pull it open.

It wasn't long before Dr. Santos came in. He was a short, dark-haired man in his late fifties or maybe early sixties, very easygoing and jovial. He was a friendly, patient-hugging type of doctor, and he talked a lot. You could easily imagine him wearing a Hawaiian-print shirt and shorts underneath his medical smock, or on his days off.

Dr. Santos told Andréa to lie back. Then he put gloves on and performed an internal exam, as Liz, Erica, and I all looked away. The entire time he was talking nonstop. "Everything looks really good," he told Andréa. "You're healthy and good to go. Given your history and my exam, I believe it shouldn't take long." Then he added, "But I usually run blood tests, which I'd like you to have."

We'd been hoping that Dr. Santos would perform an insemination this cycle, since Andréa had recently had her period. She would be ovulating soon, and Liz and Erica had already picked out their frozen donor sperm. We were disappointed when he wanted to wait for the test results to come back.

Dr. Santos ordered all sorts of blood tests for Andréa. As we left the office to go next door to the lab, we realized that all the nurses knew Liz and Erica. The two women received many hugs as we left, all wishing them good luck. Clearly, the staff had been through Liz and Erica's infertility, and was very receptive to Andréa for what she was doing for them. They were all excited—this time it seemed fail-proof. Now Liz and Erica would be mothers at last.

We went to the lab next door, where Andréa's blood was drawn, and Liz dealt with the bill for the tests. When Andréa was finished, we sat down to wait for Liz, who was talking very quietly with the lab manager. Later we found out that the blood tests cost over a thousand dollars because we were not using Andréa's insurance. At the time, we had no idea.

But we did get an inkling that something was troubling Liz after we'd left the lab and were all standing outside by the fountain (which would become our meeting place). She looked at Andréa questioningly. "I wonder if you really need all these tests. I mean, he's treating you as if you're infertile."

"Well, he is used to dealing with infertile people," Erica reminded her.

"But there's nothing wrong with Andréa, and besides, she's only thirty." Liz was sounding frustrated, but she had already taken care of the bill. "Next time, if he orders more tests, I'm going to handle this differently," she reiterated.

Unfortunately, at this time, Dr. Santos did not order what would later prove to be the most important test of all—on Andréa's hormone levels.

Space Age Container of Goo!
May 15, 2012

Andréa had now had her second period since we'd removed the IUD. It was very short, only two days, which she thought was odd, but we weren't overly concerned. We didn't want to wait another month before insemination.

We gave Erica and Liz an option: "If you'd like, we can do a trial run, and maybe we'll get lucky and not need Dr. Santos at all," I texted Erica. She was always eager, and without wasting a moment, she got on the phone with the sperm bank. She had the sperm ordered from southern California within an hour, and we scheduled a time to come to their house for the at-home insemination.

Again, Andréa and I researched the procedure. How could we make it most effective? We watched countless videos of inseminations. At-home insemination is usually done using an oral-medicine syringe, but it looked messy and like there would be a lot of waste of that expensive sperm. *Okay, we can do this. I mean, we've done some pretty crazy things already*, I thought, remembering our salad-tong IUD removal. We knew that it would work better if we used the medical syringe with a catheter, like the doctors use. We actually found them for sale online, but they would take two weeks to get to us. I needed something with a very thin straw, but I couldn't think of what. I wandered around the house, scanning each room for possibilities, when I finally went into the bathroom and there it was! I was staring down at an empty spray bottle, with its very thin tube in the middle.

"I've found the perfect solution!" I yelled to Andréa. I took the straw out of the hair-spray bottle and placed it on the tight end of the medicine syringe (before you say anything, I did boil the hair-spray tube) and...voilà, it worked perfectly! There would be no wasted goo.

The next day, Andréa and I arrived at Liz and Erica's house for our first "unofficial" insemination. We were a little surprised as Carmen led us to an upscale three-story condominium complex.

"If they make that much money, why on earth do they live in a condo?" I wondered aloud.

Andréa quickly came to their defense. "Well, it's probably very expensive to live in Silicon Valley, babe." But I knew she wondered as well.

We parked in guest parking across from a small pool. Then we walked up to the door, which was crammed next to a garage, and rang the bell.

We stood there and waited for a few minutes. No one came, so we rang the bell again. "They are expecting us, right?" I asked Andréa.

"Yes," she replied, in a tone that made me think she was wondering if perhaps they had forgotten our important meeting.

Minutes later, we heard loud footsteps, and Liz opened the door. She seemed out of breath. "Erica is walking the dog," she said right away and gave us a rushed hug. We entered into the foyer, which really wasn't a foyer at all, but the bottom of a staircase. We followed Liz up what seemed like an eternity of steep stairs.

At the top of the stairs we walked into the living/dining room. It had new wood flooring and was furnished with ornate pieces in brown, tan, and cream. Expensive artwork hung on the walls and crystal figurines and trinkets were displayed on glass end tables. The room wrapped around a large, recently remodeled kitchen that took up almost half the space.

"There are two bedrooms upstairs," Liz explained nervously.

My early misgivings suddenly resurfaced. What was really going on with Liz and Erica? *All those stairs, two small bedrooms and expensive breakable nick-nacks? Doesn't seem like they are planning on having a baby!*

As if she were reading our minds, Liz said, "We'll be moving into a bigger house when the baby comes, and Brittany will be moving out."

Soon we heard Erica bustling up the stairs and saw a little tan, long-haired dog leading the way. We gave Erica a hug. It was a relief to see her, and she seemed much more relaxed than Liz.

"Did Liz give you a tour?" she asked, and began pointing to the different areas of the room. As she pointed toward the kitchen, we noticed a tall, narrow box covered in FedEx labels. "That's it," she said as she took us over to the box. It was already open, and we could see a metal container inside, which looked like a space-age cylinder with a tightly latched top. "That's the sperm in there," Erica explained.

We were surprised that it came packaged like this, but then again, I didn't know what we were expecting.

"Wait until you see this," she went on. She unhooked the top and cold smoke immediately leaked out from underneath the lid.

"Holy smokes, is it going to blow?" I joked. "This thing is intimidating."

She reached for a little white handle and pulled out a long stick. "Don't touch the sides," she warned us. "They'll burn you." Secured to the end of the stick was a small, thin vial. It was only about one inch long, so small you could easily miss seeing it. "This is it," she told us, "This little bit cost over six hundred dollars."

We had the feeling that Liz and Erica were in a hurry, because within a matter of minutes after we'd arrived, we were preparing the frozen sperm. It could live for only a few minutes after it was thawed.

After carefully popping the vial off the end of the stick, Erica gave us a step-by-step demonstration of how to thaw the little swimmers. First she placed some water in a bowl and zapped it in the microwave for a few seconds. She used a thermometer to test the temperature of the water. As soon as it read 98.6 degrees, she dropped the vial of goo in. Erica was clearly an old pro at this.

Erica offered us a glass of wine while we waited for the frozen sperm to thaw.

"This could be it!" she said, rubbing her hands together excitedly.

I took my homemade inseminator out of my backpack and showed the girls my invention.

"That looks exactly like what they use." Liz was impressed. "You should patent that." Within minutes, the translucent white liquid, which ended up being no more than a tiny drop, was thawed, and Erica suctioned it up into my handy inseminator. We discussed the logistics and decided we should perform the "procedure" in their bedroom. Liz and Erica led the way, and then left us alone in their room so that I could help Andréa. I would call them to come up when Andréa was ready.

Earlier, Andréa and I had talked about it. We knew Liz and Erica would want to push the syringe to release the swimmers, so they would have the feeling that they were the ones who impregnated Andréa with their little bundle of joy. But to my surprise, Andréa was uncomfortable about being partially naked in front of them. She gave a heavy sigh as she unbuckled her belt, unzipped, and began pulling down her jeans. Erica had left a plush towel on the bed, and Andréa positioned herself near it.

"Help me with the pillow," she said to me as she was arranging a pillow underneath her butt. "Gravity helps the swimmers head in the right direction," she explained.

I inserted the syringe into her so that all Liz and Erica had to do was push the plunger, which relieved Andréa a little.

I gave Andréa one last chance. "It's not too late to back out, Panda." She smiled and I knew it was no use. We gave each other a quick kiss, and I went to the door to call Liz and Erica.

"Hey, cover me up," she shrieked. The towel was still on the end of the bed, and I turned around and quickly laid it over Andréa's lap just as they were coming up the stairs. Once again, my sex-kitten partner was proving just how shy she really was.

"Babe, sooner or later they're going to have to see your vagi—I mean va-jay-jay," I whispered. "And soon they'll *really* be seeing your va-jay-jay, honey."

We giggled, but Andréa gave me a heavy "get this over with" sigh as both women came into the room. They seemed even more nervous than Andréa. They had already decided Erica would be the lucky one to push the syringe that was dangling out of Andréa's va-jay-jay from under the towel. They stood next to each other as Erica leaned over and gently grabbed the syringe; she looked lovingly at her wife. They both had tears in their eyes. Liz held onto Erica's arm as she pushed in the plunger. It was done. Maybe this was it.

Soon the women stepped out, and I told Andréa to put her derrière in the air. As she swung her legs up, out came a loud noise.

"Did you just fart?" I asked her. Andréa started laughing, and more sounds came out of her va-jay-jay.

"You put too much air in the syringe," she replied, and then we were both laughing and even more sounds emerged. "Ssshhh...they will hear!" Andréa said.

Twenty minutes later, we were on our way back home. We were all keeping our fingers crossed and hoping this was it.

About a week later, Andréa got her period.

Money Is No Object
June 27, 2012

Spring turned into summer. At times, the heat became unbearable in our new-old house that had no air-conditioning. I noticed that the green hills were slowly turning brown, and the air was becoming hotter as we made our drive down to Los Gatos to see Dr. Santos the second time.

"We'll do this officially, the right way," I was thinking out loud as I drove. "None of us really expected the at-home try to work, Panda." Andréa was still a little worried, as she texted Erica on the way.

"Honestly, it doesn't usually happen on the first in-office insemination, let alone an at-home one," Erica texted back.

I read the texts aloud to Andréa. "Dr. Santos's it is, then!"

We all soon found ourselves back in Dr. Santos's examination room, laughing and excited. Within minutes the doctor came in. "All the blood tests are back and everything looks good," he told us right away.

But he wanted to speed things up. He had developed his own very successful fertility regimen, and he thought Andréa should follow it. She was to start taking the fertility drug Clomid to produce more egg follicles, Arixtra (a daily injection of a blood thinner in the abdomen), and, once ovulation was imminent, a "trigger shot" (hCG) in the butt. "This will increase our chances and hopefully get you pregnant sooner," he explained.

Dr. Santos continued to have no concern over the expenses, all of which were coming out of Liz and Erica's pockets and stressing Liz out even further. The four of us left his office and went straight to the pharmacy for more costly prescriptions. While we waited, Liz was grumbling to Erica about money, and I was grumbling to Andréa about the injections. I knew how terrified she was of them, but she insisted she was willing to do whatever it took. I felt like the injections were overkill.

Why is Dr. Santos prescribing all these fertility drugs? Does Andréa really need them? Is he just trying to make money?

Soon Andréa and I were on our way home with bags of ammunition to achieve our big goal. I had given in, but not happily. "Let's go ahead and get this over with then," was my skeptical attitude.

The next morning, I tried to give Andréa her injection, but she was so jumpy and nervous that I had to give up. She was going to have to do them herself. Consequently, every morning for the next few weeks, Andréa spent half an hour in the bathroom, working up the courage to stick the needle into her stomach.

Two weeks later, we knew Andréa's body was close to ovulation. We found ourselves back in Dr. Santos's office so that he could check the progress of her egg follicles on an ultrasound machine.

This time, we were led into a different room. Because of a large ultrasound machine, it was even more cramped than the exam room had been. Andréa stretched out on the table, and it wasn't long before Dr. Santos came in and began the examination.

By now, Andréa's stomach was black and blue from the injections, which I pointed out to Liz and Erica.

"That's normal," Erica told us unsympathetically. She was speaking from her own experience with fertility injections in the past.

Normal, my ass! I was less than thrilled with her response. It wasn't her belly that was bruised now. *And weren't you supposed to pay Andréa if she had to take injections?* I didn't say anything, because I knew Andréa would be livid at me if I brought it up to them when Liz was already stressed out about money.

As soon as Dr. Santos's ultrasound wand touched Andréa's belly, he became jubilant at what he saw on the screen. "There are eight egg follicles, and two, maybe three of them are viable and mature," he said. "This is really good news," he continued enthusiastically. "Everything looks really good."

Maybe I just had a suspicious mind, but I got the distinct impression that Dr. Santos was pleased to have an easy feather to pin in his cap. He would certainly list it as a success, even though Andréa didn't have fertility problems. He told us to give Andréa her hCG "trigger" shot to prompt her body to release the eggs. We were to make the eighty-mile trek back and forth in the morning for an insemination.

The trigger shot was not a small needle by any means. It looked more like a crocheting needle. Needless to say, I was nervous about sticking this spear into poor Andréa's little tush.

Erica then volunteered, saying, "Oh, I've done it a bunch of times." So we decided to head over to Liz and Erica's.

That night we found ourselves in their kitchen, with Andréa leaning over the counter with her pants down, and Erica inspecting her very adorable derrière.

"Ouch!" Andréa yelped when the needle went in. She gave me a quick look of pain. We left soon after, with Andréa sporting a black-and-blue bottom to match her black-and-blue belly.

The next morning, we all met at the fountain outside of Dr. Santos's office again. This time we were certain it would work. Dr. Santos came in, jaunty as ever, and seemed to think so too.

"Maybe we'll get lucky and do this on the first insemination," Erica said excitedly.

Back in the examination room, we waited as a nurse thawed the swimmers and then checked under a microscope to make sure they were viable.

Within minutes, she had come back in and inserted the medical syringe filled with the goo into Andréa's uterus. Liz and Erica were at the foot of the examination table. This time, Liz was the one pushing the plunger, with Erica hugging her from behind.

They both cried. It was touching to see tough Liz become emotional over the creation of their child. Everything seemed to come together perfectly. We all felt this was it for sure.

Andréa got her period a week later.

Off to the Races, Again
July 21, 2012

Andréa texted Erica the morning she woke up with her period. She said to me, "This is so hard, babe." She looked like she wanted to cry.

I tried to make her feel better. "Panda, we knew it would be almost impossible to be successful on just one official try."

Luckily, Erica was just as encouraging. She texted back, "Well, we knew it would probably take a few times."

And off to the races we went, repeating all the steps we had taken a month earlier, and doubling the costs for Liz and Erica. Only this time, Dr. Santos decided to run another blood test on Andréa, a progesterone-level test.

Lo and behold, the test revealed that Andréa's body wasn't producing enough progesterone to sustain a pregnancy.

You have to be kidding me! He ran all those blood tests except this one?

Dr. Santos called in a prescription of progesterone suppositories for her to take.

Discouraged, Andréa and I researched online, where we stumbled upon many discussion forums of women who had experienced low progesterone and other hormonal imbalances after removing their IUDs. Apparently, the phenomenon was well known, only we were not aware of it. Many women were complaining that they went through periods of infertility after the removal of their IUDs. Some had success with progesterone supplements.

"At least now we can fix this problem," I said to Andréa, and we went and picked up the progesterone. It was $175! Up until that point, we had not asked for any reimbursement for gas or other costs we'd incurred, but this time, I told Andréa that we'd have to ask Liz and Erica to pay for the prescription. Andréa texted Erica, who paid Andréa back right away, but Erica also told her that they had leftover progesterone from the times they were trying to get pregnant and would give us theirs in the future.

Andréa immediately started putting the progesterone suppositories up her va-jay-jay, which oozed out translucent, squishy balls throughout the day and wasn't exactly an aphrodisiac. Andréa continued with the rest of Dr. Santos's fertility regimen, and her belly got even more black and blue.

Finally, it was time for us to see what Andréa's egg follicles were looking like again. This time, though, we felt even more encouraged. "Second time's a charm," I told Andréa, as we were driving to the next ultrasound appointment. The odds for success were much better, and Dr. Santos was just as encouraging when he saw what was on the ultrasound screen.

"You have three mature egg follicles, with a close possible fourth, and our timing couldn't have been better," Dr. Santos told us.

We did the trigger shot and came back the next morning for insemination, just as we had a month earlier. Afterward, we stood outside at the fountain saying our goodbyes and chatting. The four of us really felt like this was it!

"With four mature follicles, are you girls ready for twins or triplets?" I joked. I knew that Andréa had no intention of terminating unless her life was at risk. I warned Liz and Erica, "Andréa isn't one to terminate, so you might be stuck with three!" We all laughed and were happy.

Then Andréa and I left for a Vegas vacation, just the two of us. I think Liz and Erica were worried something might happen on our trip, so we made sure they were okay with it.

But a week later, Andréa got her period, early, very early.

This time she did cry.

CHAPTER 7

Carrying that Weight

August 2012

"LOOK AT ALL THE MONEY THEY'VE SPENT. I PROMISED to make their dreams come true, and it isn't happening," Andréa said, sobbing. Her guilt was unbearable, as if it were all her fault. I tried to console her, but it was no use. She could not be comforted, and I understood.

Andréa texted Erica immediately and waited for Erica's reply with worried sadness. Erica left Andréa hanging and did not text back for days.

"We will try next month," was all that Erica finally managed to say. Her reply was kind enough, though she was obviously very disappointed, but it sounded a little distant all the same.

We were all sad, but for Andréa, this was when her distress slowly started to build momentum. I began to urge her to give up.

"This is too stressful for you, Panda. You need to think about quitting," I entreated her. "Or at least get out of their wallet. It's not your money, and they chose to use it this way," I tried to reason with her.

Andréa sighed. "It's so hard when Liz is obviously so stressed out about it," she said.

Over the next few days, Andréa and I sat at the kitchen table to go over our monthly bills. Although we weren't even close to what Liz and Erica were spending, we were having a lot of out-of-pocket expenses trying to get pregnant for them. There were the long drives to Los Gatos (up to four times a month), pricy prenatal vitamins, ovulation predictors, and pregnancy tests that were all starting to add up. Andréa was nonchalant about the expenses, but I felt differently. We had recently moved into our new house and emptied most of our savings account for moving expenses. The house needed a lot of work just to make it livable.

"I don't want to spend any more of our money trying to get pregnant for Liz and Erica," I told Andréa.

She responded with an excuse: "Well, the initial retainer they paid does cover our expenses."

"Even though it does, Panda, that retainer wasn't supposed to go toward our expenses to get pregnant."

But Andréa was a closed door; she continued to defend Liz, Erica, and their wallet.

"I told them I was fertile. I feel like we should be paying them back Dr. Santos's fees because it's taking so long for me to get pregnant." She paused and thought about it a second. "We just can't ask them to reimburse our costs."

After a ten-minute debate, I decided to let it go. I wasn't going to change her mind.

Throughout the next few weeks, I subtly continued to urge her to quit. Andréa countered that she had signed on for six months, and then she had verbally agreed to continue until the end of the year, and she would do just that. She wouldn't go back on her word.

Why is this so important to her? I couldn't help but wonder.

There were a few times when she muttered that she felt God was paying her back. I naïvely assumed she was referring to her naughty teenage days, when she gave her parents a lot of angst. I was going to find out that I should never assume anything.

One night Andréa and I were lying in bed talking, as we always did.

"Babe, maybe they aren't supposed to be parents," I told Andréa. "Why are you carrying this weight? Why do you feel that not getting pregnant is *your* karma? Why is it not *their* karma?" I asked.

I was trying to make sense to Andréa; I didn't expect her to have a real answer. But she did, and I was caught off guard.

Andréa wore a nervous smile as she bit her upper lip, contemplating my questions. Then I saw tears beginning to flow down her face. Just as soon as the awkward smile had come, it was gone. "You don't understand," she said almost inaudibly.

"What don't I understand?" I asked her gently, realizing there was in fact more to her desire to be a surrogate. I wasn't at all sure that I wanted to hear what she was about to say, but I knew I had to.

Andréa began talking through tears as she started to explain to me a secret she had been carrying—a secret from her past. It was causing her overwhelming guilt, and it was why she was so adamant about being a surrogate for Liz and Erica. She was trying to right a wrong.

Andréa had had a late-term abortion that she never got over emotionally.

Her guilt was tremendous. She had already been quite a few weeks along before she realized she was pregnant and then because of scheduling conflicts, she had to wait to have the procedure done on the very last legal day possible.

She tried desperately to make me understand. "It was a terrible thing for me to do, but I felt I had to." She described her life at the time, reliving the pain. She had already had Jared, and Julianna was only a few months old. She was financially supporting her violent, alcoholic husband, even though she was in the process of leaving him. She didn't love him. She was working twelve-hour graveyard shifts to keep the family going, only to come home in the morning exhausted and have to watch the two babies during the day while she tried not to fall asleep. Meanwhile, he slept all day and then stole money from her wallet and the kids' piggy banks to buy beer. It was no life.

She knew that if she had the baby, she would not only trap herself further into that horrible life, but also Jared, Julianna, and the new baby.

She knew what she had to do, but as the years passed, she never forgave herself for doing it.

"I feel like if I create and give this life to Liz and Erica, I'll be in some way righting that horrible thing I did," she explained to me, still sobbing.

I was shocked and hurt that she hadn't been honest upfront, but I couldn't be mad, especially when she was crying. If anyone understood shame and keeping skeletons in the closet, it was me. Even though I was disappointed, I just stroked her arm and let her know I loved her. I did wonder, though, *Is there anything else she's hiding?*

Andréa continued to pour her heart out to me: "Now not only am I not giving back that life, I'm breaking Liz's and Erica's hearts," she said, weeping.

I felt terrible seeing her in this much pain.

Red Rover, Red Rover, Let Keston Take Over!

Andréa's guilt was getting worse and worse; Erica's heart was breaking; Liz was becoming more and more frazzled over the money they were spending; and I had the overwhelming feeling that I needed to fix this and make everything better for everyone—really for Andréa. She and I were always each other's champions. It was breaking my heart to see what she was going through.

Up until this point, I had been a quiet participant. But now I knew something had to be done. My mind was consumed and spinning. *I have to get out of the passenger seat and take over the wheel. I have to help Andréa make Liz and Erica's dream come true.* I was on a new mission.

I began researching on the Internet like a crazy person, typing in one search after another in my quest for answers.

Some interesting bits of information began repeatedly turning up. I discovered that while some women's fertility and cycles never return to normal after their IUDs are removed, most settle down in time.

Well, that would have been nice for us to know. In time? How much time?

The more research I did, the more clearly the IUD was implicated as the cause of Andréa's fertility problems. Her periods were sporadic and her cycles were short, sometimes with heavy bleeding and other times with almost no bleeding at all. We were aware, from the blood tests, that she was having progesterone-level problems.

Andréa had begun tracking her body temperatures for ovulation patterns. I immediately had her stop taking Dr. Santos's remedies to start a more natural course. We began with a healthy diet, fresh air, and natural supplements, instead of all those high-powered chemicals.

Then my research revealed that frozen (outrageously expensive) sperm loses a lot of the "swimmers" in the freezing-and-thawing process. I talked to Andréa, Liz, and Erica about the possibility of using "fresh" sperm at home—meaning using the turkey-baster method with a hired anonymous donor. I found a website of donors (who had all been medically tested), and, knowing that Liz wanted the baby to look somewhat like her, I picked out attractive Middle Eastern men and sent their links to Liz and Erica.

This was a small relief to Andréa. "At least we can stop spending Liz and Erica's money," she said with hope.

Liz agreed and asked how we could reach out to these men. Erica did not respond. She seemed to have given up. Liz seemed to be taking over on their end as well.

Over the next few days, I registered on websites for local fresh donors, but we didn't get any responses. I texted Liz to give her an update while talking with Andréa about our next step.

"Well, we know some Middle Eastern men. Can we ask them?" Andréa wondered. We did, but none of them were willing to donate.

Liz decided the baby didn't need to be Middle Eastern after all. That opened up a whole new set of possibilities.

As we texted, Erica started to get involved again, and that made Andréa very happy. Erica's enthusiasm began to revive. She and Liz even asked whether my son Zack or any of his friends might be interested, since they lived in our basement.

Liz joked, maybe half-seriously, "What a shame, when there's all that fresh sperm downstairs from you."

Yuck! The thought grossed me out, as amusing as it was. We left the subject at that. I didn't want to be Zack's creepy upstairs mom asking the boys for something as outrageous as this. We weren't that desperate—*yet.*

We were in limbo for a few weeks until Andréa and I received a text from Erica that would be another game-changer.

Enter Shawn and Rod
August 30, 2012

Andréa and I were at a diner eating breakfast one morning when a text from Erica came through. She read it to me as if she were Erica speaking: "How do you feel about using sperm from a friend of ours?" A second later, another text popped up from Erica: "An at-home insemination."

For a moment, Andréa and I were both quiet as we took in this idea.

"Geez, Panda, I don't know if I'm comfortable with that," I said doubtfully. Andréa nodded in agreement as she bit her lip in deep thought. I continued, "We don't know if the sperm is clean. We don't know if it's disease-free. At least the donors from the donor site have all been tested."

I sighed, knowing Andréa's silence indicated she was more open than I to this plan.

I hesitated, and then asked, "Who are they thinking about using?"

Andréa immediately looked down at her cell phone and began typing to Erica, "Who do you have in mind?"

"Our friend Shawn; you've met him," Erica replied.

We barely remembered Shawn. We had very briefly met him and his partner Rod when we went with Liz and Erica to an amusement park. "Shawn seemed nice," Andréa said, softening to the idea.

"But are they disease-free?"

All of a sudden, I heard my mother pop into my mind as if she'd magically appeared in the empty seat at the table. Mom would have had a field day with this one!

"He probably has that gay disease," she said scathingly. She would not have let that one go. She wouldn't have even remotely tried to be politically correct. She believed that most gay men had AIDS. I tried many times when she was alive to educate her, but she was strongly opinionated.

"Andréa can get it. The baby could have it. Can't you find a normal *man?"* Mom nagged inside my head.

"I hear you, Ma. I promise we won't do anything stupid," I assured her silently. Her presence faded as I turned and spoke to Andréa. "He has to be tested. Andréa, he could have AIDS, for all we know."

"It's not going to cost Liz and Erica anything at all," she reasoned with me. "Liz won't be so stressed out about money anymore, and I won't feel as pressured."

We were not at all on the same page, but this time, I wasn't going to budge. "Andréa, I put my foot down. No. Not unless we know he's tested."

I told her to text Erica and explain that Shawn needed to be tested, and she did.

"Yes, both Shawn and Rod have recently been tested and are clean," Erica responded immediately, as if she had been waiting for our question.

I rolled my eyes as Andréa read Erica's response to me. *Just recently, huh? Well, that's mighty suspicious.* But Andréa's smile grew even bigger as she read Erica's next text to me, as if she were gloating.

"Shawn and Rod recently decided to have a baby and use their own surrogate to get pregnant, so Shawn has already gone through a thorough medical checkup," Andréa read.

Of course, I was still suspicious. While Erica's response cleared up my health concerns, it did prompt another flaming-red flag for me.

By now we had left the diner and were driving home. Instead of dictating to Andréa, I took advantage of our being stopped at a traffic light; I picked up my phone and texted Erica myself, repeating out loud for Andréa as I texted, "How do you know they won't want to keep the baby if their surrogate doesn't come through for them?"

"They would never do that. Our agreement is that they will be uncles. That's all they want. They will have a baby of their own." Erica sounded certain.

Well, I guess that would be Liz and Erica's problem. Not ours. I knew I had to let it go.

Andréa decided she was okay with Shawn donating. Since he had recently been tested, I once again supported her decision. She texted Erica to tell her she was willing to go through with it.

Erica planned our next move. She asked Andréa to let her know when she would be ovulating so that she could arrange the at-home insemination. We knew it was coming very soon. We would have to drive to Shawn's house in Gilroy when it was time.

Andréa thought she would be ovulating on Erica's birthday, and sure enough, a week later the prediction test indicated she was. Andréa texted Erica, telling her that she had a positive ovulation test.

A few hours later, Erica texted back, "Rod wants to donate too. Is that okay?" She added, "This way it will be more anonymous."

Andréa didn't see a problem with it, but it made me feel weird. I muttered, "That seems dirty."

Andréa glanced at me with a disgusted look on her face, obviously annoyed at my ignorance. "Well, I'm not having sex with them! What does it matter? It just increases our chances."

Oh, my God, what she will go through to help these two!

And so our trips to Shawn and Rod's house in Gilroy began.

Old MacShawn Had a Farm, E-I-E-I-O!
September 8, 2012

Two days later, we found ourselves driving south. Summer was coming to an end, and the air was still warm. Our drive down to Gilroy was boring and long as we passed the now tan-and-brown hills in the East

Bay, then flat, industrial San Jose, and finally entered farmland. I was excited, though. I would be getting my fall decorations out when we got back home.

We had an additional forty-five minutes to go, making the round trip just less than four hours. Because we wanted to do two donations back-to-back, we planned on spending the night at Shawn and Rod's.

Erica had warned us that "the boys" lived "on a farm," so I was surprised when Carmen stopped us in front of a typical 1980s suburban home in the middle of a neighborhood.

This isn't a farm! What in the world was Erica talking about?

Liz and Erica arrived right behind us, and we were grateful to walk in together. Neither Andréa nor I felt quite comfortable with any of this.

An attractive man of average build with longish sandy-brown wavy hair, piercing blue eyes, and a fresh shave opened the door. It was Shawn. Like Liz, he obviously cared about his appearance. Wearing a tailored button-down shirt and designer jeans, he looked like he belonged on the cover of a romance novel.

Pretty good-looking guy, I thought.

Erica reintroduced us, and we shook hands. I wasn't surprised when Shawn spoke with a subtle gay lisp. He was animated and used his hands much like Erica did.

His older husband Rod, an African-American man, emerged from their kitchen to greet us. He was taller than Shawn, but just as attractive, with a five o'clock shadow that seemed as though it was planned. He was clearly a body builder with broad shoulders, a thick neck, and ripped biceps that made his arms protrude. While not as animated as Shawn, Rod also had subtle high-pitched tones in his voice.

Both guys seemed nice enough.

Considering their different appearances, I immediately thought the baby wouldn't turn out to be so anonymous. "If the baby comes out with dark features, it'll be obvious," I whispered to Andréa as we were given a tour of Shawn and Rod's house.

"The baby will be beautiful either way," Andréa whispered back.

The first stop led us to the backyard, and there I understood why Erica had called their house a farm. Shawn had turned their large yard into a mini farm. Chicken coops and cages lined the exterior fence lines, and roaming around the beautifully manicured lawn were several varieties of chickens, rabbits, and ducks that were being chased by two barking dogs.

Then we went inside the house, where more exotic animals lived—colorful birds, snakes, fish, and turtles in almost every room.

Okay, so these dudes are eccentric! I snickered to myself.

I had brought wine and cherry vodka for Andréa. Erica had brought beer. She poured all of our drinks as Liz cooked Mexican food. As I looked around the room, I noticed pictures of Shawn at a much younger age, posing with exotic animals, mainly elephants and tigers.

"I used to be a zoo keeper," Shawn explained, as he pointed to the many pictures.

In no time, dinner was ready, and we ate the delicious carne asada Liz had prepared. As we ate, we were all talking and trying to get to know one another, pretending we weren't nervous about the purpose of our visit. Once we were finished eating, Shawn did the dishes. I didn't want to open another bottle of wine, so I had one of Erica's beers.

Erica must have felt Andréa's anxiety over the upcoming insemination. "Well, should we get this done?" she suggested as she stood up, rubbing her hands together. There was no need to ask what she was talking about.

She got a unanimous yes. We all wanted to get the deed out of the way.

After spending a few minutes searching for the perfect vessel for the specimen, Shawn found a miniature martini glass, which he amusingly thought would fit the bill. The guys marched upstairs to obtain their donations.

Awkward! Andréa and I gave each other a look.

"This is weird," I admitted as Liz, Erica, Andréa, and I waited downstairs.

Erica agreed. "Nothing we've done is normal, but I feel good about this. It's my birthday, after all."

We all felt like maybe this was the magic night.

About fifteen minutes later, the men came downstairs with their martini glass and its white goopy contents.

Yuck! From the looks on the other women's faces, I felt like all four of us had the same thought. But we had to do what we had to do. I pulled my syringe invention out of my backpack and gave it to Liz. At first, it looked like she was about to hand the cute little martini glass to me.

"Oh, no, no. I don't want to touch it," I teased her, and made her keep the glass as the four of us went upstairs. Liz headed straight into a small bathroom to fill the syringe over a sink, while Erica stood outside the door watching. Around the corner, Andréa and I were getting her ready in the guestroom where we were to stay for the night.

The room was painted a dark red and decorated with blatant appreciation for the male body. There were statues, plaques, and paintings of male body parts everywhere.

"Some guest room!" I laughed as Andréa and I looked around.

Andréa was in position with a pillow under her rear end and a towel draped over her lap. I opened the door and Liz came in and handed me the syringe, which I quickly inserted into Andréa.

"It's ready," I told Liz and Erica.

Since it was her birthday, Erica leaned down and squeezed the plunger. Then all four of us began talking nervously, hoping the yucky goo was doing its magic.

"You should see what's in this closet!" Erica waved her hand toward the corner of the room.

I had to oblige her and opened the closet door for a peek. As soon as I saw the feather boas and handcuffs, I closed the door as fast as I had opened it.

Oh, I shouldn't be looking at this. More weird, weird, weird! But I admit that I was amused.

Soon enough, we were all back downstairs sitting around the dining room table.

Erica had an emotional moment: "Look how lucky I am that I have four people on my birthday doing this huge thing for me." We all felt that the magic mojo of the birthday gods would shine down on Erica, and we would finally get pregnant.

Shawn and Rod kept talking about someone they called "Li-Lo," as if this person were some sort of celebrity. Eventually I realized they were referring to Liz!

Good Lord, these gay boys have a lesbian crush!

We spent the night so we could do another insemination in the morning.

A few weeks later, Andréa got her period.

Hope Was on Its Way! But Was It Lost?
September 26, 2012

Although it was agonizing, it didn't come as a surprise to Andréa or me that she had gotten her period. We had been tracking her temperature charts, and it appeared that once again, she had not ovulated. She broke the news to Erica. We were becoming accustomed to it, but it still hurt every time. This time, though, it involved six of us instead of four. To make matters worse, Andréa's cousin Janelle, who was unmarried and still living at home, announced that she was pregnant. Janelle had been close to Erica when Erica had dated Kris.

Andréa still carried the weight of her failure. "I promised them I would give them a baby," she said sadly when she came out of the bathroom after discovering that she got her period.

Each time, she cried and felt overwhelmed with guilt. I felt bad too, but I tried to soften the blow. "Maybe Liz and Erica aren't meant to be parents, Panda," I said again as I washed dishes in the kitchen.

Andréa leaned against the wall, staring down at the floor, defeated.

This month was even harder, because Andréa had promised me we would give up at the end of the year, which was fast approaching. She had told Erica the same thing.

"Can't you fix this?" Andréa looked up at me pleadingly, half joking but with tears welling up in her eyes. "You always fix everything, Keston." It was true; I usually did fix everything for her, as she did for me.

I felt as if a ton of bricks was falling on me; this was a huge challenge. I knew Andréa wasn't serious, but I did take her seriously.

"Panda, I'm not a doctor." I paused and thought while I dried my hands. I gave her an uneasy smile. "But let me see what I can do."

"No, babe, I was just joking. You're not a magician." Andréa looked beaten. "I know you can't fix this."

Or can I? I'm not a person who can be told I can't do something. This would be a challenge, but I was going to try.

I would refer to my tried-and-true holy grail of information: I went online. For days, I researched: sitting on the couch, at the dinner table, in bed, pulling up every website I could find on fertility problems. I barely ate; I barely showered. I was a crazed woman. Andréa quietly let me be.

I need to be Andréa's hero. I need to fix this. I was obsessed!

I began by troubleshooting the facts. *Okay, we know Andréa isn't producing enough progesterone. Her cycles are still short. From tracking her temperature, we know she's having cycles of anovulation* (meaning that she wasn't ovulating normally), *and we strongly suspect the IUD seriously compromised Andréa's hormones.* I read countless threads, message boards, case studies, and marketing scams.

One late Monday evening, I stumbled upon a thread on a message board on which women with similar problems were talking about their successes and failures. One woman posted that she had been trying for three years to get pregnant after having an IUD, when a midwife told her to use an herbal supplement, a berry extract called Vitex. This woman posted that after years of trying, she had been on Vitex for only two months before she got pregnant! I kept reading, and felt that I might be onto something.

This might be it! I was excited, but it was late. I knew that if I kept exploring this new subject, I'd be up all night, so I went to bed. I would start researching in the morning.

For some inexplicable reason, I have a totally reliable internal alarm clock, no matter what. Even when I'm super tired and have gone to bed late, I still can't sleep past 6:00 a.m. The night of my discovery was to be double trouble for me, as I was so anxious to check out this "magic" herb. I was like a kid on Christmas Eve. By 6:15 the next morning, I was up in the dark with a cup of coffee and my laptop at the kitchen table, and back online.

It was as if I had opened Pandora's Box. There was page after page of stories about Vitex and its success helping women with hormonal imbalances get pregnant.

Where do I buy this? And how expensive is it? I found it (where else?) on Amazon. It was forty-five dollars a bottle, plus ten dollars for shipping. And there were hundreds of reviews, mostly four and five stars. *Eureka!* I was ecstatic.

Andréa was still asleep, but I was so thrilled I decided to wake her up. I sneaked in and leaned down to kiss her.

"What are you going to give me if I fix this?" I whispered. She moaned, pulled a pillow over her head, and gently pushed me away. I lifted up the pillow and asked again with more authority, "What are you going to give me if I can fix this?"

Andréa knew exactly what I was referring to. She started to stretch, but didn't open her eyes.

"Mmmmm. Babe, you know I was kidding. You're not a doctor." She reached for the pillow, which I had tossed aside.

For the third time, I repeated my question: "I said, what are you going to give me if I can fix this?"

Andréa opened one eye first and then both, blinking at me. She knew I was serious. I would never have awakened her so early otherwise. After a few seconds, she took a deep breath and then said, "Um, how about we take five hundred dollars from our first payment, and you get to choose whatever you want to do for a date night?"

"Sold! I can fix this!" I proclaimed without a second's hesitation, and a deal was struck.

I went on to tell her about Vitex.

Andréa was skeptical. "I don't know. That is a lot of money for just one month of pills," she said.

"It's worth a try," I insisted. And off I went back to my laptop to order the herbal pills. I was secretly worried, though. I'd read that while some women got pregnant right away, typically it took three months for Vitex to be effective.

Do we have three more months?

I paid an extra twelve dollars for rapid shipping, and the Vitex arrived five days later in a small brown box that had "Amazon" and a smiley mouth printed on it.

I opened the bottle as fast as I could and handed Andréa a pill.

We noticed right away that her cycles and body temperature began normalizing. It was looking very promising. Now Andréa wasn't so skeptical. I saw a new sparkle in her eye, as if her faith was returning. But I had a lot on my shoulders if this failed. *Holy shit, I hope this works!*

If at First You Don't Succeed
October 5, 2012

After a few more weeks, we did a second insemination with Shawn and Rod's goop. It worried me that we were doing it too soon. I felt that the Vitex needed at least another month to work. This time, we decided not to spend the night. Andréa and I would just come back the next morning.

During this visit, Shawn informed me that their surrogate had started her period. "I was so upset that I hung up on her," he told me. He added, "She just got divorced and has a new boyfriend whom she's having lots of sex with."

I had no idea what to say, but I managed, "Yikes, how are you going to know you are the daddies?"

"I know, right?" Shawn said, his hands in constant motion as usual. "Well, we can't complain, since we aren't paying her."

You're kidding me!

"Is she your sister?" I paused, "or a family member?" I couldn't believe anyone in her right mind would do this for free, even though I believe Andréa would have had I not forced the issue.

"No, just a good person and a good friend," he responded, raising his eyebrows at me, as if I needed to read between the lines.

Later, when Liz, Erica, Andréa, and I were up in the guest room performing our insemination, I probed Erica for more information. I was wondering how she felt about Shawn and Rod's surrogate arrangement. Perhaps they now felt that Andréa should be doing this solely out of the goodness of her heart as well?

Erica was more than happy to get into the gossip of it all. "Oh, my God, can you believe that?" she said, to my relief. When I repeated what I had said to Shawn about not knowing whether their baby would be theirs or their surrogate's boyfriend's, she kept nodding and saying, "I know." She told us that the woman was from Alaska, and she was infatuated with Shawn. "If you ask me, I think she wants some type of threesome family relationship," Erica said as Liz listened and nodded.

"There's no way that's going to happen. Rod has never even seen a vagina, let alone been with a woman." Liz grinned mischievously and shook her head over how grossed out Rod would be.

Up until this point, after each insemination, we had all been hopeful and excited. When I told Liz and Erica about Vitex, they did not seem as encouraged as I was. But who could blame them?

"This time," we used to say, "is the one!" But now, we were almost inured to the disappointment, and we all seemed to be just going through the motions, especially Erica. I don't know whether Liz was just trying to encourage Erica or whether she herself still had hope. At any rate, she was much more vocal and positive than before. None of us was quite ready to give up yet.

We parted hoping, but not expecting.

Even though they were becoming much more stable and consistent, Andréa's hormones must have still been out of whack. Although she and I knew from her body temperatures that she was not ovulating at the time of this latest insemination, it still hurt tremendously when two weeks later she got her period again.

I was hoping Liz and Erica would give the Vitex time. *Be patient.*

Hope is on its way. I couldn't help having a deep conviction that the Vitex would work if we could only give it two more months.

Poor Erica, it seemed like she wanted to give up, but just couldn't let go of her dream. She was so sad. The four of us discussed the plan and decided to stay on track until the end of the year. That would be only two more tries.

I ordered a second bottle of Vitex, which arrived just in time for the next month.

CHAPTER 8
Third Time Is a Charm?

October 27, 2012

IT WAS THE SATURDAY BEFORE HALLOWEEN. THIS TIME, Shawn and Rod could do only a one-shot donation, and only on that Saturday afternoon, which was a few days early for Andréa's ovulation day. They were too busy with Halloween parties.

When we arrived at the men's house, Liz and Erica were already there. An awkward silence greeted us as we entered. I was overwhelmed by a peculiar feeling that our arrival had interrupted a deep conversation the four of them had been having about us, and that whatever had been said wasn't nice.

The air was tense with hostility toward Andréa and me, but mostly toward Andréa.

Without enthusiasm, Erica said flatly, "October is our lucky month," as if she were just being polite. I followed her as she walked outside onto the backyard deck and sat down in a deck chair. She wasn't even pretending to be friendly.

Liz was again more upbeat than usual. I thought she was concerned about Erica's depression. She reminded Erica, "We met in October, got married in October, et cetera," encouraging Erica to believe that indeed October was their lucky month.

Andréa and I gave each other a "things feel odd" look, reading each other's minds. We were feeling hopeful, though, and we weren't going to let their resentment dampen our spirits. We saw that the Vitex seemed to be working, and for the first time in months, Andréa's temperatures indicated that she was ovulating more normally.

While my heart was excited, I couldn't help being angry with them. *How dare they?* But rationally, I understood their frustration. I let go of my anger as best as I could.

Andréa hurried upstairs to get ready, but as if admitting defeat, Erica looked at Liz. "You do it. I'm going to stay here." She wouldn't let herself get involved any more. Liz could push the syringe by herself this time.

Liz followed Andréa, but I felt like I needed to stay with Erica, who had not moved from her deck chair. I sat down next to her, feeling sorry for her. I also felt protective of Andréa. It was awkward, and I was filled with a nervous energy.

Should I try to cheer her up? Maybe I'd only be setting her up for another heartbreaking letdown.

I tried to spark a conversation with the first words that popped to mind: "Did you read on Facebook that Janelle is pregnant?" As soon as the words left my mouth, I realized that was a horrible topic. *Damn it, Keston!*

Erica looked bewildered. "You're fucking kidding me," she said with a raised, angry voice. "Does she still live at home? Is she married? Didn't she just start dating this guy?"

"Yes, no, and yes," I responded, wishing I'd kept my big mouth shut.

"I guess *anyone* can get pregnant," Erica said sarcastically. She was shaking her head disbelievingly with her hands up in the air, as if she were asking God why.

I was grateful Andréa wasn't around to hear the implicit criticism that was almost certainly directed at her. But I realized that I probably asked for it.

There was a long, awkward moment of silence.

"Hey, if October is your lucky month, girl, maybe you should go upstairs with Liz to push the syringe," I urged Erica.

She was quiet and stared straight ahead, in deep thought. "You're right," she sighed, and then got up and headed upstairs.

Only a few minutes later, Shawn and Rod came out onto the deck after shooting their deposits into the martini glass, and I found myself still sitting in the same chair, but now with Shawn in Erica's seat.

"Our surrogate backed out," he told me abruptly.

Red flag, red flag!

I told him I was very sorry to hear that.

In a mean tone, he added, "Again, we can't complain." His hands were waving around in the air. "We weren't paying her," he sneered, emphasizing the word *paying*.

Ouch! And I see that worked well for you! I was shocked at his directness. It was clear that Liz, Erica, Shawn, and Rod were, in fact, talking about Andréa and me when we arrived. And it was pretty obvious that there was some resentment toward us.

I thought Shawn's comments were extremely inappropriate, especially since, other than the initial retainer, Andréa had not yet received any compensation. Furthermore, we hadn't even asked for reimbursement for our own costs. Feeling surer than ever that this time the Vitex would work, I bit my lip and chose to ignore Shawn's comment.

Within minutes, Andréa came back downstairs, and Shawn propelled us to the door almost as soon as she had reached the bottom step. "Sorry, but we have to go. We have a party to get ready for."

Liz and Erica were standing next to him. There was no small talk. We hugged quickly and walked out the door. Liz and Erica stayed behind.

I don't remember Rod even speaking to us at all that day.

Andréa and I got in the car and stared at each other, not exactly sure what to say. But we had a mission of our own, and Andréa didn't want to waste any time. "Drive around the corner and find a parking place quick!" she directed me.

I knew what she wanted.

"There is no place to do this, Andréa. You are going to have to forget it," I said with conviction.

"We are going to have to do it in the back of the truck," Andréa insisted.

"No way, it's broad daylight. Everyone will see us and it's a hundred degrees in here," I pleaded to Andréa's common sense. At that moment, she had none.

She had recently read that having an orgasm made the cervix open so that the tadpoles were more likely to get where they needed to go. She'd prepared me for her request the week before, but at the time, I didn't realize the logistics involved.

"You agreed," she said, now getting angry.

"Now, Panda, just where do you expect this to happen?"

"I don't care. It just needs to be done, and done now."

Grumbling, I knew it was no use fighting, but I could still complain, "You're not going to be the one with your ass sticking up in the air!" I protested, knowing Andréa needed to lie flat so the swimmers wouldn't seep out.

She wasn't going to give up. My arguing was futile. I knew what I had to do. The longer I put it off, the more frustrated with me she would get.

I drove around corners and up streets, but I couldn't find a secluded place to park. "It has to be done *now*!" Andréa was getting agitated.

"Okay, okay." I parked the truck right then and there across from a park. "Thank God we brought our Explorer and not the little Lancer." I laughed, trying to make things lighter to set a nicer mood as we climbed into the back.

Andréa started taking off her jeans with her feet in the air. Even though it was October, it was hot as hell in the back of that truck.

I tried to assert my authority as I started sweating. "I'm keeping my clothes on."

"Okay, but unzip your pants." I agreed to the compromise and we got busy!

After I gave Andréa what she wanted, we hit the road, finally able to talk freely about how we'd just been treated at Shawn and Rod's.

"You felt it too, like they must have been talking about us?" Andréa said.

"Oh, yeah, and it really bothers me. We've done an awful lot for them." I didn't elaborate on my conversations with Erica and Shawn. I knew it would hurt Andréa's feelings. "You could have given up long ago. At least you're still in it to win it, all for them."

"I don't understand why they'd be resentful. This isn't costing them more money, and I told them I'd give it until the end of the year." She looked sadly out the window. "They don't appreciate what I'm doing for them."

Now I was able to be angry. Lucky thing that they never made their snide comments to Andréa's face; I might have said things to protect her that I would have regretted later. To tell the truth, I would have loved to tell them exactly what I thought, but it would not have been a great idea. It wasn't the time for that, but I looked at them differently now.

"You can't do this again, Andréa. They're not grateful," I told her sadly.

I was surprised that Andréa did not make excuses or argue. She nodded, and together we decided on the drive home that if it didn't work this time, we were finished. This was going to be our last try.

Andréa was at peace with it.

Bad Timing
October 28, 2012

The next morning over breakfast, Andréa and I talked about our chances of pregnancy in the coming month. We weren't too hopeful. Ovulation occurs two to three days after a positive test and we hadn't gotten one until that morning.

"It was just too early," Andréa reflected. "That's a really long time for the swimmers to wait up there for the egg to arrive, and they could only do one shot. I'm almost certain we'll miss my ovulation window. It would be a miracle if it happened." She paused. "And it will look like my fault again."

I just sat there listening to her pain. I didn't know what to say.

After the coldness we'd experienced the day before, I really didn't care anymore. Eventually I spoke up. "We agreed, Panda, this was the last time."

Andréa nodded. "Yes, but we can still make this window if we get another donation."

Oh, my God! I put my head in my hands.

She saw my frustration. "Look, I promise this will be the last month. But it kills me knowing I've let Liz and Erica down, Keston. If this is the last month I can try to make their dream come true, let's give it our all."

I gave in with a compromise: "I love you and I will support you, but only if I have your word that this really is the last month."

"After the way they treated us yesterday, I can make that promise." Andréa's tone was certain. The clock was ticking. If it didn't happen this month, it would not be happening at all.

Andréa finished breakfast and texted Liz and Erica about her concerns over missing her ovulation day.

Liz was the one to respond, not Erica, which was unusual. "Shawn and Rod are just not available. Would one of the boys downstairs be interested?" Her first text was followed by another: "Maybe we pay them something?"

Ugh! Although we had definite grossed-out feelings about this prospect, we were more desperate and open to the idea than we had been before. And the more Liz texted about it, the more she seemed to like the idea. "The good thing about other donors is we'll never know who the biological father is," she texted.

"I don't know if any of them would do it," I texted back. "I'll check. I'm sure it would have to be a hundred percent anonymous."

Time to Give Up
November 5, 2012

Over the next week, Andréa's temperatures seemed even more regular, but they did not rise and fall in a pattern consistent with pregnancy. We were sad, but this time, it was different. We were both somewhat relieved.

It was time to move on.

After multiple months and six insemination attempts, the effort was just wearing too heavily on everyone. I had to protect Andréa. I couldn't bear to see her anguish over this any longer, and I believed she wanted her torment to stop as well. We were going to get off this roller coaster.

"The Vitex really needed that third month. Your cycles are much more normal, but it says that it typically takes three months," I told Andréa. Nevertheless, after the snub we had gotten from Liz, Erica, Shawn, and Rod, we weren't willing to give it another try, even though we had initially agreed to continue through December. This time there was no argument. Andréa agreed.

"I'm going to wait to tell Liz and Erica until I officially get my period, though," she insisted. Andréa hated any form of confrontation, especially giving bad news. Every time she had to tell Liz and Erica she'd gotten her period, she did so promptly, but it was very hard for her. This time she would not only have to tell them she wasn't pregnant, but that we were quitting.

"Just get it over with," I told her. "We already know your temperatures aren't consistent with being pregnant."

"After the last time, I don't have the heart to tell them, Keston. I'll just wait until I get my period and tell them like I always do," she insisted.

Over the next week, we kept busy, immersing ourselves in the renovation of our house. We had already remodeled the kitchen and were now starting to work on the basement. I was knocking down walls, putting up walls, and replacing floors, while Andréa rewired the electricity and added outlets. It was a nice change of pace for us. Andréa looked surprisingly sexy in a white tank top, oversize men's cotton boxers, and a backward hat, along with a pink leather tool belt I had bought for her.

"Ya know, now that I'm not pregnant or trying to get pregnant, I think I want to be an electrician's apprentice," she told me. I thought she would be great at it.

It was going on a few weeks after our last Gilroy trip when Liz texted Andréa, asking her to take an early pregnancy test. Andréa looked up and bit her lip as she read Liz's text. Then she said, "Oh, God, I don't feel like telling them again that I'm not pregnant."

"Just get it over with, Panda. You're procrastinating."

Andréa sighed. "No, the plan was to wait until I get my period, so I'll stick to it." She texted Liz back, "It's still too early." Liz seemed to understand, and we went back to work.

"Strange, though, that your period hasn't started yet," I thought out loud.

Andréa shrugged. "Just another unpredictable cycle."

A few days later, I realized again that it was odd that her period still hadn't started. "Maybe just for shits and giggles you should go ahead and take a pregnancy test."

"No, I can't bear to, because then I would have to tell Liz and Erica I'm not pregnant."

A few more days passed.

Liz texted again, "Take an early pregnancy test."

"Not yet, it's still too early," Andréa replied.

I knew she tended to procrastinate, but this time she was holding out even longer than usual. "Babe, what's the difference whether you just tell them your temps indicate you're not pregnant, or you go take the damn pregnancy test? Sooner or later you have to tell them." I was getting frustrated. "Besides, why hasn't your period started? We need to rule out pregnancy and find out what's happening to your body."

"There's no way. My temps aren't consistent enough," she insisted.

I think we were both intrigued, but neither of us would admit it. I was insistent. "Either way, you should take the test. Suppose something's wrong, and we should have you see a doctor?" I added, "Just humor me."

Andréa shook her head stubbornly and refused to do anything.

"Geez Louise, Panda, you can't avoid telling them for much longer. You'll get your period soon either way, and if you don't because something's wrong with you, then you're giving them false hope." I uttered my final words on the subject and gave up, as Andréa appeared to ignore me.

But I must have said something that struck a chord.

The very next morning I was sitting on the couch reading Facebook when Andréa came out of the bathroom. She was visibly shaking and holding a thin white stick in her hand.

It was a pregnancy test with two dark-red lines. It was positive!

CHAPTER 9

Positively Wonderful!

November 11, 2012

I JUMPED UP FROM THE COUCH AND RAN OVER TO
Andréa as fast as I could. She held the test up for me to see. The two red
lines on the stick weren't even remotely faded; they were as dark as they
could get. Andréa was shaking so hard, she couldn't talk.

"Holy shit!" I yelled. We danced around the room for a few minutes.
"How are you going to tell the mamas?" I asked her.

She was finally able to speak, but her voice was trembling. "They'll
still be asleep. I won't say a word. I'll just send them a picture of the
positive test." Andréa had already thought it out. She was laughing and
crying as she took a picture of the test, and then she texted the photo to
the girls without adding a word.

We were so excited, we couldn't think or talk about anything else. We
imagined Liz and Erica waking up and opening the picture. "It might take
them a minute to realize what it is," I laughed. "Erica is going to cry."

"She's been dreaming of this moment for so many years." Andréa was smiling through the tears in her eyes. And now it was finally happening. It was real. It was awesome! We were caught up in the prospect of Erica's joy.

It was hard to wait for them to wake up. Andréa was so excited, she was downright slap-happy. "They'd better get all the sleep they can now, because sleeping until 10:00 a.m. isn't going to be an option soon!"

We stayed close to Andréa's phone the rest of that morning. It seemed as if Liz and Erica would never wake up. Finally, a few hours later, the phone rang. It was Liz.

They had us on speakerphone. There were long periods of silence when they were so elated they could barely speak. "Is this real?" Erica kept asking. We assured her that it was.

They were interrupting each other as they told us how they had opened Andréa's text and realized what it was. Liz was awake before Erica and saw the text first. She woke Erica up with two words: "Andréa's pregnant."

Erica thought Liz was playing a cruel joke on her. "I told Liz, 'Don't fuck with me,'" she said, imitating the nasty tone she had used.

We were all laughing and crying as Andréa and I reassured her. "Yes, it's real!" I yelled.

"Your dream is coming true," Andréa chimed in.

And Andréa is their hero! Andréa is righting that wrong! I thought as I smiled over at my beautiful partner.

"You don't understand," Erica chimed in. "Just yesterday, we got some very bad baby news about our adoption that fell through."

We had no idea what she was talking about, and we were taken aback.

"The timing couldn't be better," Liz started to explain. Just two weeks earlier, right around the time we had our last insemination, they had been chosen to adopt a baby boy. Then yesterday, they had found out that the adoption was denied. They were heartbroken. They had already paid for the adoption, made a nursery, bought baby-boy clothes, and thought it was a done deal.

Andréa and I were stunned. It hurt that they had kept us in the dark while they went ahead with adoption plans.

What about Andréa? Geez, what would they have done if they got that baby and this baby too?

It was shocking, but Andréa and I were too excited to hold a grudge for long. We were all so happy, it didn't matter. Andréa had done it! Everything was glorious!

The next few months were a celebration—except that Andréa was sicker than she had ever been in her life.

A Peanut by Any Other Name
November 13, 2012

Liz and Erica left it up to Andréa to choose an OB/GYN who would take her insurance. After quite a bit of research, we found Dr. Rose, who had recently moved to the Bay Area from Florida. He had excellent reviews and was in Walnut Creek, so Liz and Erica wouldn't have to drive all the way to Antioch. It would save them about thirty minutes of travel time when they came for the baby's appointments. And it was conveniently located across the street from the hospital.

Andréa coordinated her first appointment with Liz and Erica's schedules.

We all met in Dr. Rose's tiny waiting room. It accommodated only five patients, so the four of us almost filled it. We squeezed into the little white space and sat down on the teal floral-print couch and the two tan armchairs at each end.

As we waited for Andréa to be called, Erica handed Andréa an envelope. It was her first payment since the retainer.

The door opened and a nurse called Andréa's name. When all four of us stood up and prepared to follow Andréa in, the nurse looked confused.

"Andréa has three wives," I joked, trying to ease the unusual situation. She still looked confused, but she didn't say anything.

After taking Andréa's weight and blood pressure, the nurse handed her a white paper gown and told her to get undressed. Still looking bemused, the nurse left us.

A few minutes later, there was a light knock, and a stocky man with dark features peeked in. "Hello," he said in a friendly way. I was surprised Dr. Rose was so young, maybe thirty, but we instantly liked him. He had a genuinely nice smile, a soft voice, and a great bedside manner. He seemed like a boy-next-door sort of guy.

This time Erica took charge of clarifying why four women would be coming to Andréa's appointments. "Andréa is kind enough to be having our baby for us," she explained, and then briefly described our surrogacy arrangement. Dr. Rose was more supportive than we could have ever hoped. He even told us that he had grown up in a house full of women, so all the estrogen in the room was a nonissue for him.

He was excited about his new high-tech ultrasound machine. As he moved the wand over Andréa's belly, he pointed to a small circle on the monitor and exclaimed, "That's it! The fetal pole!" For the first time, we saw the little black ball that was Liz and Erica's baby. It was surreal to actually see the result of our months of efforts right there live on the screen. Erica and Liz held hands.

I started to get teary too when Erica, who was crying, leaned down to get a better look at the screen. "There is our Peanut," she said, and then looked up at Liz, who was equally emotional.

"According to the size of the baby, your date of conception was October 31st, which will make your due date July 21st." Dr. Rose was thinking aloud while he wrote down his notes.

Seeing the baby this soon had us so excited that we almost forgot to talk to Dr. Rose about Andréa's morning sickness. We remembered just in time, and he gave her a prescription for it.

We went our separate ways. Liz and Erica left with the first pictures of their Peanut in tow. It was a very happy day!

On our drive home, Andréa opened the envelope that Erica had handed her and looked puzzled.

"It's five hundred dollars short." She glanced over at me, and then she dismissed it. "Oh, well, it's never been about the money. I'm sure they'll catch up next month. I know they're good for it."

I thought it was odd. "But they know how much they're supposed to pay you. We all have copies of the agreement. Shit, Andréa, it may not be about the money, but what about the principle?"

If they make so much money, why are they shortchanging Andréa? Seriously, look at what the hell she's doing for them! Are they having money troubles?

Though we weren't overly concerned, it seemed to me that this was something else Andréa's kindness was making excuses for. *Was this another red flag?* But we were still too happy, so I let it go.

We sat at the dinner table that night discussing what we would do with the money. We were finished with major renovations on the house, and Andréa's car was still running okay, so we decided to put half the money in savings for our beach wedding and use the other half for a vacation. We would fly to Florida, buy an old, drivable RV there, and starting at Disney World, take the kids on a cross-country trip.

Morning Sickness or Death
November 29, 2012

Everything was going along smoothly, with the exception of Andréa's extreme morning sickness. "I didn't have it nearly as bad as this with Jared or Julianna," she kept repeating wanly.

It was the end of November when we went back to Dr. Rose for a follow-up appointment. As I always did, I stood behind Andréa, holding her hand as we all looked at Dr. Rose's new ultrasound monitor to see Liz and Erica's "Peanut." The baby was growing perfectly and starting to take the shape of a little person.

Now I was more concerned with Andréa's morning sickness than I had been before. It was getting much worse and had even sent her to the hospital for IV rehydration. She was losing weight and was almost bedridden from nausea. Dr. Rose decided to put her on a stronger medication. He told us Andréa's hCG levels were very high.

"I'm sorry you're so sick, but that's music to my ears," Erica said. She was relieved every time we spoke about the morning sickness. We all agreed it was a good sign that the pregnancy was strong and the baby was healthy.

Outside at our cars, we stopped to talk. I remembered reading that very high hCG was the first indication of twins. We joked about it. Had Dr. Rose's tip-top ultrasound machine missed a twin? We had also learned that higher hCG levels made morning sickness more severe. Somewhere in my research, it mentioned that it could also indicate an abnormality in the pregnancy, a statement I completely ignored.

One Big Happy Family!
December 2, 2012

We invited Liz and Erica to Jared's seventh birthday party. Tutu and Boppi were going to be there, and it was important for them to accept that Liz and Erica were firmly onboard with bringing their child, whom we were now calling Peanut, to family events.

Liz and Erica must have felt similarly. They RSVP'd at once.

When the birthday night came, Liz and Erica fit right in with the family. They played their parts perfectly and spoke openly about how, next year, they would be bringing their baby with them. They spent quite a bit of time getting to know Boppi and Tutu better, and for the first time, we were able to recount the agonizing stories of our pregnancy journey. Only somehow, now, in the retelling, all the heartache and failures seemed humorous.

I was never one to deny my curiosity, and I badly wanted to know something. After a few cocktails, I asked Erica what had happened with Shawn and Rod's surrogate.

Erica was more than happy to spill the very entertaining beans.

"She came and wanted to do the insemination the old-fashioned way." Erica raised her eyebrows humorously. "Rod was disgusted. I mean, he's never even seen a vagina, let alone gotten up close and personal with one!" Andréa and I grinned, and Erica was laughing so hard, her words came out in a rush: "So Rod wouldn't do it, but Shawn put the syringe up there, but then he must have taken it out too fast, because it was all coming back out, and Shawn had to push it back in with his fingers!"

We all collapsed in hysterics as we imagined Rod's face during this fiasco.

Liz finished Erica's story: "Rod was horrified."

She went on to say that the surrogate seemed to have wanted some sort of two-father, one-mother arrangement, with everyone living together as one big, happy family. When she realized that wasn't going to happen, she decided not to be a surrogate for them, Erica told us.

My Date Night from Hell
December 8, 2012

Fall had turned into winter without our even noticing. Thanksgiving had passed. The air was now cool, although it would never get too cold. The tan colors were gone from the hills, which were now almost entirely a dull brown. My pilgrim decorations were back in their boxes, and a Santa statue I had painted for Mom when I was ten was now in their place.

As she'd promised, Andréa agreed to let me plan our five hundred dollar date night. I had always wanted to go to the Dickens Fair, which was held every Christmas season, so I planned our date around the fair right after Thanksgiving. We would also have a nice dinner and a romantic stay at the Embassy Suites by the bay.

Liz and Erica told us they wanted to contribute too, so they watched the kids for us that night.

We checked into the hotel, and off to the Dickens Fair we went. It was always at the Cow Palace, a huge event warehouse south of San Francisco.

As soon as we pulled into the parking lot, we felt underdressed and much too modern. Many people wore antique English costumes. We entered the fair door through heavy curtains, and felt as if we'd been transported back in time. Inside was a fantasy old English village, complete with half-timbered shop fronts, inn and tavern signs, and fake shipping docks. We got there in the late morning, but inside the lighting was dim, as if we were strolling through an old England town at night.

There were wonderful smells everywhere—of roasting chestnuts, soaps, lotions, cookies, and hot chocolate. Other than Coca-Cola, everything the vendors peddled was authentic to old England. They were selling mulled wines, ales, bangers with mash, meat pies, and fish and chips. The stores had handmade crafts, old English attire, soaps, pewter candlesticks, very old books, dishes and jugs, and Christmas ornaments.

The fair had a magical feeling!

From Scrooge himself to a bearded lady, and even the patrons, everyone stayed in character. I was mesmerized and just wanted to melt into it all. I thought about having English ale, but decided I didn't want to be sleepy and miss anything. And there was still the rest of our date and dinner later, so I stuck with the thick, delicious hot chocolate.

This was my day, so I got to choose everything we ate or did—that was the deal. "What should we have for lunch?" I excitedly asked Andréa. "I know! Bangers and mash!"

"Whatever you want, babe, it's your date." Andréa smiled at me with an uninterested look. She was strangely pale.

Just as we got in line to order our lunch, she suddenly gasped, "I don't feel good. I have to find a bathroom now." She ran from the line.

I tried to catch up with her as she was darting through the crowd. "Stop, babe!" I yelled. She turned around. Her pale face had a green tinge to it. At that point, I realized just how crowded the facility was. "This place is like a huge maze." I was getting nervous as I tried to read the map we'd been given. It was hand-drawn and hard to read, but I felt I could make some sense of it as I started leading Andréa through the crowds. We had to find a bathroom. After skirting past hundreds of people, bumping into the (very solid) Ghost of Christmas Past, and working our way around a crowd watching a statue of a chimneysweep come to life, we finally found a big burgundy curtain with a sign on it that read "Privy." We went through the curtain and found ourselves outside in a large circle of Port-a-Pottys.

Oh, man, Port-a-Pottys? "Hurry, there's an empty one!" I yelled and opened the door as fast as I could for Andréa to stagger inside.

Within seconds, horrible, gut-wrenching sounds were coming out. I couldn't imagine that the smells in there were making Andréa feel any better!

People were looking suspiciously at me, like Andréa was some young, drunk girl. "She's pregnant," I kept saying. I stood outside for about half an hour waiting for her to finish. She finally reemerged, still looking very pale.

"We have to go." Her voice had a serious tone.

"What? But we just got here," I whined as if I were a child.

Andréa looked at me ashen-faced, as if she could scarcely see me. "I have to lie down."

I knew she couldn't help it, and I didn't want her to feel bad, so I hid my reluctance and disappointment. "Okay, we'll come back next year. Anyway, I think the kids will love this. We'll bring them too. You owe me a do-over for next year!" To that Andréa agreed, looking sorrowful, and we left only an hour after we had arrived.

We went back to the hotel. We didn't end up having dinner, nor did we have time for any romance. I had a really bland and unmemorable room-service meal and watched a movie by myself while Andréa spent most of the night on the bathroom floor.

A Flicker of Hope
December 11, 2012

At the third obstetrics appointment in mid-December, the four of us met again in the waiting room. Erica handed Andréa another envelope, December's payment.

We were all thrilled to see Peanut again on the ultrasound. Everything was looking perfect. It was amazing to see the baby's growth. This time, I saw a flicker on the monitor.

"Is that the baby's heartbeat?" I asked, but I already knew. Dr. Rose confirmed it. Liz and Erica were watching, transfixed, with tears in their eyes, as we all followed the flicker of light beating on the monitor.

At the end of the appointment, Dr. Rose had a question.

"Between eleven and fourteen weeks gestation we offer an in-depth ultrasound called a Nuchal Translucency scan. It can detect abnormalities by measuring the collection of fluid under the skin at the back of your baby's neck. Would you guys want to do that?" Realizing that he may have alarmed us, he quickly added, "I don't expect any abnormalities here. This looks to be a normal, healthy pregnancy, but many people choose to go ahead and do the scan."

"That's up to the mamas," Andréa said, pointing toward Liz and Erica.

They turned to each other for a moment, talking quietly. Then Erica said, "Another ultrasound? We can see our Peanut up close and personal? Why not?"

And with that, Dr. Rose's nurse scheduled the NT scan for a little over three weeks away. We left his office and walked out together, eager for the next visit.

"Even on the very slim chance something was wrong, we wouldn't care," Liz said.

We could hardly wait to see Peanut up on the screen in high definition. We started counting down the days!

Once again as we headed home, Andréa opened the envelope Erica had given her.

"It's five hundred dollars short this time too," she said, looking at me. Not only had they failed to make up for their first short payment, but once more, they had underpaid Andréa. And we weren't talking by just a little bit.

"Should I say something?" I frowned.

"Hmmm…maybe they're just waiting until the baby's here to catch up completely, but that kind of bugs me. Shouldn't they ask me if that's okay?"

"Yes, of course they should," I said. I couldn't understand it.

"It kind of sucks, I mean, I'm clearly going through a lot for them."
But in typical Andréa fashion, when it came to Liz and Erica, she came
up with another excuse: "I'm sure they're planning on catching up at
the end."

Up Close and Personal
January 10, 2013

Christmas and New Year's Eve had come and gone. The only thing we
looked forward to now was getting to see Liz and Erica's Peanut.

I drove Andréa to meet them for the NT scan. I knew I couldn't be
in the room, since they usually allowed only one extra person and were
already making an exception for both Liz and Erica to be in there. I
would be in the waiting room for support, though. I was eager to hear
all the great news.

We met in the waiting room of the perinatal office. It was in a new
building only a block away from Dr. Rose's office and the hospital,
the John Muir Medical Center, where we were planning to have the
baby delivered. The waiting room was large enough for us all to sit
comfortably. It was a restful place, with nicely painted mauve walls and
two sections of tan leather chairs. While we waited, we admired the
poster-sized black-and-white photos of children hanging on the walls.
There was also a large flat-screen TV suspended from the ceiling. It was
tuned to a National Geographic wildlife video with Oprah Winfrey
narrating.

We sat down and talked about how exciting this detailed ultrasound
would be.

"Get them to print out a picture so I can see Peanut too," I begged
Erica.

She patted her purse and told Andréa that she had January's payment
for her just as the waiting room door swung open and the nurse called
for Andréa. I stayed behind, trying unsuccessfully to focus on Oprah

talking about flocks of birds in the Serengeti. My thoughts were certainly not on birds in Africa!

About twenty minutes later, the door to the waiting room opened. I expected to see a nurse, but it was Liz. She leaned out the door and beckoned me to come in. I was up and on my way in a second.

"They're going to let me in? I get to see?" I asked her excitedly.

Liz shook her head. "No," she said in a low voice. "There's something wrong with the baby."

CHAPTER 10

Something Wrong with the Baby

"WHERE IS ANDRÉA?" I ASKED LIZ, WITHOUT FULLY digesting what she'd just said. I felt like I was having an out-of-body experience or a bad dream as Liz led me down the hall.

This can't be happening. This is not real. What is wrong with this perfect baby?

I knew I needed to get to Andréa as fast as I could. All Liz could manage to say was "Come," and I followed her down a short hall until we entered a secondary waiting room.

This must be where they send people who have a poor diagnosis, who need privacy, I inappropriately thought.

It was decorated in the same colors as the first one. This time Oprah was talking about marine life and the animal kingdom on the big-screen TV.

Andréa was sitting in one of the tan armchairs, crying harder than I had ever seen her cry. I ran up and threw my arms around her. She clutched me and burrowed her head into my stomach. I kept holding and hugging her as hard as I could. Andréa looked up at me and I could see in her eyes what she was thinking.

No, Panda, this—whatever this is—isn't your fault! You're not being punished.

Erica was also crying and holding Andréa's hand.

Andréa looked up at me. "You should have seen Peanut, babe. Peanut is so cute."

Erica nodded, but was obviously in shock as she spoke. "The baby was moving, kicking its legs, twirling around. I couldn't believe it." Her voice was shaking.

Liz interjected, "We were joking about our little basketball player. The baby looked perfect."

I was puzzled. "So then what's wrong?" I asked.

"There's a buildup of fluid behind its neck, indicating a chromosomal abnormality." Andréa looked up at me as she spoke, tears streaming down her face.

A few minutes later, I learned that the baby had a thick nuchal translucency reading of 7.2 millimeters. The normal range was 1.0 to 3.0 millimeters.

Erica then said, "The doctor said that this is when parents choose to terminate and start over."

I was in shock and didn't know what to think or feel. My only instinct was to protect Andréa. In my typical fashion, I wanted to save her, save the day, but I was devastated and at a loss. I could only hold her and support her.

At the urging of the doctor, who had already suggested termination more than once, Erica and Liz had decided to immediately do a CVS (Chorionic Villus Sampling) test where the doctor takes cells from tiny fingerlike projections on the placenta called the chorionic villi and sends them to a lab for genetic analysis.

Another nurse came to get Andréa. This time I would be going with her. Wild horses couldn't have stopped me. Liz and Erica decided to stay in the separate waiting area. We were led back down another long hall into an ultrasound room, where the procedure would be performed.

I barely noticed the room we were put in, except for a general impression of dim lighting, soft grays, and state-of-the-art equipment.

There was a big-screen monitor on the wall directly in front of the examination table for eager parents to see their baby in high definition. Andréa was told to undress and lie on the examining table. I held her hand.

It was in this room that I met Dr. Spencer for the first time. We didn't wait long before he came in. He was tall, middle-aged and of average build—maybe in his late forties, early fifties—with a receding hairline. He combed his dark hair forward over his long forehead to conceal it. I must say that to me, he looked a little bit like a thin Frankenstein.

Dr. Spencer had a cold, matter-of-fact bedside manner and seemed slightly arrogant.

"Who are you?" he demanded, looking straight at me.

I had little patience with his curt question. I explained who I was in a direct, no-nonsense "don't fuck with me" tone. He must have taken me seriously, because he seemed a little less abrasive as he took the time to explain why he felt the baby had chromosomal abnormalities.

He said "terminate" at least three times as he told me what I assumed he had told Liz and Erica. The more I listened, the bleaker his picture became. "This is probably worse than Down syndrome."

That was when reality hit me like a brick in the face.

Down syndrome? I was shocked! *What could be worse than Down syndrome?*

"You mean retarded?" I asked in a defeated tone as I pulled my hand away from Andréa for a second and drew it up to my mouth, taking a deep breath.

"Yes," he replied. "The baby also has fluid around its heart and probably has a heart condition as well." He went on to say that the baby could be "severely deformed." He literally made us think that Peanut would turn out to be like the Elephant Man. "If you guys want, I also perform terminations, and I can schedule that today." He spoke as if he were helping us make a hotel reservation.

Andréa just lay on the table quietly crying and not saying a word. It was going too fast, and I needed things to slow down for her. My charm was out the window. "Wait. Wait a second. Could it be just a heart problem and not Down syndrome?" I asked.

"It is possible, but not likely. This baby almost certainly has chromosomal abnormalities and most likely has severe heart problems. It will probably pass away on its own." Dr. Spencer certainly had no faith beyond his machines and his own ego.

I heard "heart problems" and clung to it.

The baby has serious heart problems. That is what's happening here. I wouldn't even consider that Peanut had Down syndrome.

Dr. Spencer must have seen where my mind was going. "It's probably not just heart problems." He was grounded in his doom-and-gloom prognosis, and I still wanted to hold on to hope.

"We don't even know what's wrong with the baby. We need to know exactly what we're up against," I told him bluntly. "Let's just do the CVS and see what really is going on."

He didn't argue. He seemed like the type of man who was too busy to waste time on an argument.

He quickly went over the CVS process with Andréa. "It's an invasive procedure. It's performed by perforating your stomach with a needle into the placenta to extract DNA from the womb. It can cause a miscarriage," he told us.

Andréa nodded. I moved to the head of the examination table and stood behind Andréa with my cheek against hers.

My poor Andréa, she's so terrified of needles!

Dr. Spencer turned on the ultrasound machine to help him guide the needle. Once he pushed it through Andréa's abdomen he started jabbing and scraping her belly forcefully. I placed my hand on her heart underneath her shirt and whispered, "I got you, Panda." I pressed my lips to her ear.

But Andréa could only reply, "God is punishing me. God is going to make me kill another baby, Keston." With tears streaming down her face, she didn't seem to care who was in the room hearing her. As much as I wanted to, I could not take the pain away from her.

As Dr. Spencer was prodding and jabbing, I looked up at the

monitor and saw the same beautiful baby Liz and Erica had seen just thirty minutes before. Dr. Spencer turned up the volume and I could hear its heart.

Ta-ka-cha, ta-ka-cha, ta-ka-cha. It sounded like a strong little train.

I was amazed at what I saw. Peanut was clearly now a baby, moving its arms and kicking its legs. To me, Peanut looked perfect. But I did notice the bubble behind the baby's neck.

Could that really be so sinister?

Dr. Spencer pulled out the needle, turned off the monitor, and handed me a picture of Peanut that he had printed out. "If you pay to have the results back sooner, we can have them by Monday," he told us in his cold, businesslike way.

Liz and Erica decided to pay Dr. Spencer the extra four hundred dollars to rush the test results, but we would still have to wait until Monday. Three days was unbearably long!

The air felt heavy as we walked out of the office. We talked about our hopes that Dr. Spencer was wrong. Contemplating his worst diagnosis of Down syndrome, I told Liz and Erica that if they kept "that sort of baby" they would be better women than I. Then as quickly as I acknowledged the worst possible diagnosis, I dismissed it again.

The baby has a serious but fixable heart problem, I kept telling myself.

"Somebody doesn't want us to be mamas," Liz said, looking up toward the sky.

We were all four in tears. Now all we could do was to wait for three terrible days.

Either Erica was too heartbroken to remember, or she chose not to give Andréa the envelope containing her January 1st payment.

The Longest Wait

It was tense in the car as we drove home; neither Andréa nor I said much. I just kept repeating to myself, *the baby has heart problems. Can we fix them?* I was going to go home and research fetal heart problems. I was deliberately shutting out what Dr. Spencer had drummed into us about chromosomal abnormalities. There was just no way that this could be Down syndrome. God couldn't be so cruel. It was unthinkable, but the more I refused to believe the baby had Down syndrome, the more it pushed into the front of my mind.

We got home and Andréa immediately had to get ready to go to a meeting with Boppi for his Swiss Club, of which she was also a member. She could hardly bring herself to get ready, but she didn't want to let him down.

I talked to her as she dressed.

"Panda, this baby has serious heart problems. I don't believe the baby has Down syndrome, but clearly it's sick and is fighting for its life." I took a deep breath. "I know we agreed that you"—I took another deep breath between tears—"*we* would not get attached and would not give this baby our love while it's growing inside of you, but you have to now, Panda."

Andréa stopped getting ready and looked at me intently with welling tears.

I could not—would not—admit that this baby might have something in my mind as hideous, as grotesque, as Down syndrome. For the brief split seconds that I considered it, I pictured a drooling child hitting its head against the wall. I saw a lifetime of what my sister Rhonda had become. And I quickly dismissed that thought.

I continued explaining to Andréa my plan: "This baby needs to feel love to get it through this heart condition. Maybe with love a miracle will happen." *And it won't have Down syndrome. Maybe we can love the Down syndrome away and it will be a heart problem.*

Andréa knew me very well. She knew why I kept saying "heart problem." She looked tenderly at me and said, "Babe, love and praying aren't going to make this baby not have Down syndrome. It already has what it has."

But I still couldn't bring myself to acknowledge that we had created what in my mind was a monster. *Certainly we should be rewarded for our good deeds*, I thought. "Miracles happen, Andréa. Maybe some divine intervention will make a miracle? Either way, this baby is sick. It's fighting for its life and it needs to feel love. You're the only person who can do that."

"I know." Andréa gave me a half smile through tears, and gazed at me as if she were seeing deep into my soul. "I know," she said again.

I had to watch the kids while Andréa went with Boppi to their meeting. She told me that later that night on their drive to San Francisco, she'd told Boppi what was happening. "He was very supportive, as usual. He thinks it's too late to terminate the pregnancy," she told me. "He hopes Liz and Erica do the right thing." Somehow, it helped that Boppi felt that way.

This weekend was supposed to be my birthday weekend, but now neither of us felt like celebrating. Except for when we were taking care of Jared and Julianna, Andréa and I spent the entire weekend in tears, off and on, or else we stayed in bed doing online research. We learned everything about thick nuchal translucency measurements, how the buildup of lymphatic fluid could possibly turn into a cystic hygroma (abnormal growth filled with fluid) or hydrops, which is the deadly accumulation of fluid, and other complications that can be caused from the excess fluid.

Andréa told me of her finding that Down syndrome was called Trisomy 21. Babies with Down syndrome often have thick NT measurements because their lymphatic systems develop more slowly, but it does not necessarily turn into cystic hygroma or hydrops for them.

"Quit talking about Down syndrome! The baby doesn't have Down syndrome," I told her, not wanting to face the image of the child I had created in my imagination again.

It was a heart-wrenching three days. At times, I walked into the dining room and stared down at the picture of Peanut lying on the table. I saw what looked like a beautiful, perfect baby. I ran my finger across the ultrasound picture, remembering the bubbly personality of this little being I had seen on the monitor.

During the weekend, Andréa handed me a bag with my birthday present in it. She had bought it for me while we were still rejoicing over the baby. I opened the bag and found a small red teddy bear that sang notes of a song each time its belly was pressed. She told me that she had searched the Internet for it because the song was special to her. I tried to smile as I pressed its belly over and over so that it could sing its song.

"Let me call you sweetheart / I'm in love with you / Let me hear you whisper that you love me too."

I smiled, but I could not fathom celebrating, or even a happy red teddy bear. I had a burst of anger that we were going through this, and here I was supposed to be celebrating! I didn't want the bear and tossed it to the side. Andréa looked at me, disappointed.

Surprisingly, I didn't sense my mother being around. I don't think she would have known what to say.

As the days and hours ticked by that weekend, the more I tried to dismiss the thought that Peanut might have Down syndrome, the more it kept popping up in my head that it really might be true. I continued to talk to the baby in the ultrasound picture. A few times, I talked to God and I point-blank begged him to keep the baby from having Down syndrome. The thought just overwhelmed me with despair. It was so horrible that I couldn't bear to open up to Andréa about it. To me, there could be nothing worse on the planet! I wouldn't, couldn't accept it. I so desperately wanted this to be something else and convince myself of that, I continued searching online for what else it could possibly be.

I found some answers that seemed to be what I was looking for, but nothing more. A lot of heart conditions could be an issue, so I hooked onto that and wouldn't consider anything else. In my mind, I started moving past the diagnosis. *The baby has a heart problem; so can we fix it?* I was relieved when I felt I had enough information from my research to convince myself that, yes, I had diagnosed this as a heart problem, not Down syndrome.

I found myself again staring down at the ultrasound picture of Peanut. All of a sudden, I felt as if the baby in the picture was trying to tell me something, but I didn't know what it was. I smiled as I ran my finger across the photo again as if I were actually touching the baby. "You're just fine, little one; you're going to be a miracle. We are going to get you through this heart problem," I said aloud to Peanut's ultrasound picture, as if the baby would hear me, and God would grant a miracle.

I went back to the bedroom and picked up the smiling red teddy bear, then turned and faced Andréa, who was sitting in bed and still researching on her laptop. I spoke fiercely: "This baby is going to be fine. I'm going to play the teddy-bear song every day for the baby, and someday, Andréa, I promise, I'm going to give the baby this teddy bear." I held the bear close to Andréa's belly and started playing the song. Andréa didn't say a word. She smiled at me but was still sad. At that moment, we didn't even know whether the baby was alive.

That weekend, Andréa continued to spend countless hours researching like crazy, trying to find anything that could be the cause for the thick NT measurement. She thought that perhaps Rod was the biological donor and that Peanut had his pudgy, thick neck. She even pulled pictures off Facebook to show me the back of Rod's head. "See?" She tried to convince me. I hoped that she was right.

Finally, Monday morning came. Andréa and I chose to stay in bed. We just lay there and waited for the call. I told Andréa, "At 9:00 a.m., we're going to call Dr. Spencer. We're not sitting around all day in misery."

But we didn't have to wait that long.

The Worst Day Was the Best Day
January 14, 2013

The phone rang at 8:30 a.m. It was Dr. Spencer. This was it.

Please do not be Down syndrome. Please do not be Down syndrome.

He got straight to the point. "The baby has Trisomy 21," he said. I closed my eyes and bowed my head.

Andréa asked, "Positive for Down syndrome?"

He was blunt: "Yes."

It was out now. But I already had known deep down, because I wasn't surprised. My immediate feeling was great sadness for Peanut, who hadn't asked for any of this. *How can God do this to Peanut?*

Dr. Spencer added in a very detached tone, "And it's a girl," and shortly thereafter hung up.

"It's a girl," I said out loud. It didn't seem to matter.

I felt a familiar sickness in my stomach that I had felt only once before. It was when I realized the clawed woman in the corner of that assisted-living facility was my sister. But this time I couldn't run away. This time I couldn't fix it, and this time I couldn't call my mother.

Andréa looked up at me, tears pouring from her eyes. She gave one heartbroken bursting sob, and then picked up her phone to call Liz and Erica. This was devastating news, but we knew they were waiting, as we had been just a few minutes before.

They picked up on the first ring, and Andréa told them the results: "The baby has Down syndrome, and it's a girl."

There was silence on the other end.

"I'm sorry, we have to get off the phone and digest this." Erica sounded withdrawn. She and Liz seemed a million miles away. The four of us were not sharing this sorrow.

The air in our bedroom was heavy. This was it. It was over. I assumed we would have to schedule a termination. I looked at Andréa and felt so sad for her and Peanut.

To my amazement, she opened up the laptop, but instead of researching causes of thick NT measurements she was now researching Down syndrome. I looked at her with sadness.

What does this mean to her? She'll be terminating another baby, but this time God is taking over and making her do it. This is the wrong she's been trying to right. This is her worst nightmare come true.

Throughout that day, Andréa never put the laptop down. The kids would pop in and ask for lunch or a snack, which I got for them, but Andréa did not get out of bed. She was learning everything she could about Down syndrome, crying all the while. We didn't tell the kids what was happening, but they enjoyed their day of unusual freedom, watching movies and playing video games in the playroom we had made for them downstairs.

I paced in and out of the bedroom, often walking out to the ultrasound picture still on the dining room table and staring down at it. *I am so sorry, little one, I am so, so sorry.* I couldn't bring myself to think about her pending termination. The first thing I would have done in any normal circumstance was to call Mom. *Oh, God, Ma, I need you.* I would have to do the next-best thing and ask her to be with me. I closed my eyes and imagined her near me. Soon, I felt that Mom was there.

I could hear her, *"Oh, geez,"* breathed out in a sad, shocked tone. There would be a long pause then. Mom would not know what to say.

"What are they going to do?" she'd ask.

"There's not much they can do. I just don't know, Ma. I don't know what any of us will do." I felt helpless. There weren't any answers.

"Well, you'll just have to try again," she would respond.

"After how they treated us? I don't know if that's an option, Ma." I was looking over at Andréa as Mom's presence faded.

I was grown up now. I couldn't turn to my mother anymore. This burden was mine to carry.

Several times throughout that day, Andréa and I acknowledged to each other that we couldn't help but feel that Liz and Erica were not supposed to be mothers. We both said it several times. I had wondered about this before, when we were having such a hard time getting pregnant.

"Maybe we pushed it when we weren't supposed to?" I said. "I mean, after all they went through before, and all we went through together in the last year, to finally get here and this is the card we were dealt?"

But now, there was a baby. Even though she wasn't "perfect," she existed. She had a personality. We all saw it on the huge ultrasound screen just a few days earlier. She had a heart, a beautiful profile, and we were about to realize that she also had a fighting spirit.

Later we texted Erica and let her know we had scheduled an appointment for all four of us to go see Dr. Spencer's genetic counselor, Ms. Friedman, the next day, to go over the results.

"We should be as educated as possible," I texted.

Throughout the day, Andréa watched countless videos about babies, children, and adults with Down syndrome. She eventually asked me to come into the bedroom and watch them with her. She already knew what she was going to show me.

Do I really want to see these? I thought. But Andréa was in so much pain, how could I say no?

Andréa's Courage

I had zero desire to watch videos of disabled people, but I could deny Andréa nothing that day. She had the courage to see for herself what this meant. She wanted to find out exactly what a person with Down syndrome was like. She faced it head-on and looked at it for what it was. She was going to educate herself, and—very quietly—she was going to educate me. She did not just give in to the "termination" suggestions of Dr. Spencer. How thoughtful she was, without saying a word about her pain. She just looked weary and sorrowful as she played video after video for me.

As we watched, she never said a word, but was saying so much with her eyes and her grief. I knew from the look on her face that she did not want to terminate Peanut. She looked at me between videos, tears welling up. She wasn't narrating or explaining anything. She wanted me to see for myself. Knowing how I felt about disabilities must have made this so much harder for her. I was keenly aware that if Liz and Erica backed out, the direction Andréa and I would take would depend entirely on me. I knew how much Andréa loved me. She would do whatever I wanted to do, and she would not push me.

It was then that I realized Peanut's life or death was ultimately up to me. Just like Mom's life was, not so long ago. I had thought that I would never be put in this impossible position again, yet here I was. In my immediate mind, I could only fathom termination, but I was finding it difficult to say the word.

I couldn't save Mom back then. I knew it was hopeless, but in my heart, my role in her death was always lurking in my subconscious—always too heavy to really process. *Was it really hopeless? Or did I just give up on Mom?*

Now I was in a very similar role in another hopeless situation.

Because of my guilt over Mom's death, I couldn't make this kind of decision again before I was absolutely sure that Peanut's condition was in fact hopeless, and as I sat and watched the videos with Andréa, for the first time I was willing to acknowledge and look past my own phobia. I wanted so desperately to find hope.

As I watched the videos, I was surprised by my own reaction. I wasn't disgusted at all. I almost cannot describe how I felt, but I know I was not horrified anymore. To my further surprise, the videos showed some of the most adorable little babies I had ever seen!

"They're actually really cute," I said, acknowledging what Andréa already knew. We saw many triumphant videos where these kids had beaten the odds and survived multiple open-heart surgeries. But most important to me, the videos showed them reading and signing literally hundreds of words by the age of two. I felt hope growing in me.

I was dumbfounded. *Wait, aren't all of them supposed to be scary-looking vegetables, hitting themselves or drooling in a corner?* I saw no monsters, not even one! And there were not just a few videos, but hundreds of these kids overachieving. *How is that possible?* We watched a video about a man with Down syndrome who opened his own restaurant, and another who was a popular barista at a local coffee shop. We watched a video of a young actress with Down syndrome who had a role in a television series opposite Academy Award-winning actor Jessica Lange and is very intelligent and well spoken.

"They hold down jobs?" I was amazed. "I never knew."

We were inspired by a motivational speaker named Karen Gaffney. She has Down syndrome and had swum the English Channel. She was so eloquent and inspiring that it blew my mind.

I looked over at Andréa. "These people can do anything anyone else can do!" I was surprised. I had found my hope—the hope that I lost when I gave up on Mom. I had found it that day—the worst day, but the best day.

Something deep inside me was changing. To my complete astonishment, I heard myself say, "Peanut can make a difference, and probably more so than any 'normal' person."

But how was this possible? We learned so much that day about the monumental advances in therapies that now included ways for these children to learn, more than ever before. They were contributing members of society. So many advancements had been made since the Eighties, when they were still warehoused or institutionalized like those I had experienced.

The fact that Peanut had survived the first trimester gave us a glimpse into her feisty personality, now that we knew that up to eighty percent of miscarriages in the first months of pregnancy were due to chromosomal abnormalities like Down syndrome. If the babies did survive the first trimester and made it to the NT-scan diagnosis, nine out of ten were then terminated by their parents, based on the earnest recommendations of doctors.

"Holy shit! Peanut has already beaten some incredible odds!" I thought out loud. Andréa smiled at me, and I saw hope in her eyes when she saw a change in my face.

I felt admiration and adoration for this little fighter—and protectiveness of Peanut—welling up inside me. Eventually, I walked back out into the dining room and picked up the ultrasound picture of Peanut. I stared at it, and again I ran my hand across the little body. I now knew what the baby was trying to tell me earlier.

"You are not a monster," I said to Peanut in the picture.

And in that moment I realized, *it was me.* I was the monster. Not this little baby, not the disabled people I had come across in my life. It was me all along.

You see, in the three days since I told Andréa that she needed to love this baby who was fighting for her life, I too had fallen in love.

CHAPTER 11

And My Small Heart Grew Three Sizes that Day!

January 14, 2013

I DIDN'T HAVE TO ASK ANDRÉA HOW SHE FELT. I ALREADY knew. I came and sat next to her on the bed. She closed the laptop and then turned to look at me with her red, swollen eyes. I knew she did not want to terminate this baby whom we'd worked so hard to create, and who was made with such purpose, but she would if I wanted her to.

But I loved this baby. I didn't want to terminate her. I didn't want to take away her chances to make it. Peanut had made it so far already. She was an underdog, and she deserved a fair shot to live. I had never been more certain of anything in my whole life.

I knew what Andréa needed to hear. But could I get the words out? They came out easily: "If Liz and Erica do not want her, we can keep her. We can do this." I was trying to hold back tears.

Those two sentences with just sixteen words were magic to Andréa's ears. She gasped a crying laugh that turned into a smile. Her lip quivered and she quickly bit it.

She had to make sure.

"Keston, you don't mean that. I know how you feel about people like Peanut," she questioned me searchingly. I could hear hope in her voice.

I looked her straight in the eye. I wasn't crying anymore. I was stern and I was certain. "Yes, yes, I do mean it. Yes, and everything will be fine." I don't know why, but I had no doubt. Like Andréa, I now knew too.

She burst out crying again, even harder than before, but it was different. She was crying because her suffering had found the relief she most needed; she was crying because, no matter what, together we would save this baby and be its champions; and she was crying because she was proud of me.

We hugged for a long time. When we finally drew apart, I saw that the look on her face had completely changed from utter sadness to happiness. She smiled, and from that moment on, continued smiling.

Now let's hope Liz and Erica are on the same page with us. But it almost didn't matter anymore whether they were. Andréa and I wondered what they were thinking. We hoped that they would be Peanut's champions too. We hoped they still loved and wanted their daughter.

"Should we send them links to these videos?" I asked her.

"No, it would seem like we're trying to push them into wanting her. If they have to be pushed into loving her, they shouldn't have her." This was the first time I saw Andréa's mama bear coming out.

We would be Peanut's champions even if nobody else would! We would fight that fight with her and for her. We hoped and prayed it would not come to that. We hoped and prayed that her intended mothers still loved her.

With all the emotion and drama of the morning, I started to get a headache. I realized that I hadn't had my daily cup of coffee yet. It was now almost evening. I left Andréa watching videos and walked to the kitchen to get a cup before my headache got worse.

I had a nagging feeling as I was pouring my cup. I turned around and I could feel Mom there with me. She was not chuckling in amusement at my shenanigans. This time, she was serious.

"Keston, have you lost your mind?" Mom's voice in my head was harsh.

Mom very well might have used the word imbecile if she were around—a word I'd heard her use throughout my life. I'd even heard her use the word just before she passed away, when she was talking about VP nominee Sarah Palin's son Trig, who had Down syndrome. Mom may not have been politically correct or delicate, but she would have wanted me to hear this.

Knowing how she was pro-choice and how she felt about "imbeciles," this was a no-brainer! I think this was the first time I realized that, had abortion been legal in 1966 as it is today, I'm positive I wouldn't be here. I myself was a much-unplanned, late-in-life pregnancy for Mom. She already had too much on her plate, and she was going through a divorce from my father, who was an irresponsible nightclub singer/bartender. Maybe if abortion been legal in her day, she might have been able to live her dreams as an actress in Hollywood.

At that moment, I understood her, and I understood me. I smiled.

Usually when Mom had disagreed with me, I would question myself. But now, for the first time in my life, I would come out of her shadow without wavering.

I love you, Mom, but you're wrong.

In that moment, I gave myself permission to be a better woman.

Mumbo Jumbo
January 15, 2013

I can't say we were excited to be going to the genetic counselor, but Andréa and I at least were glad to be getting some more answers. We also knew it would be a heavy day, seeing Liz and Erica for the first time since the diagnosis.

When we arrived at Dr. Spencer's waiting room, Liz and Erica were already there. Neither Andréa nor I knew exactly what to say, but we had to break the ice.

I immediately walked up to Erica. "I am so ashamed of what I said the last time I saw you." I hugged her.

"What did you say?" she asked.

"What I said about you two being better women than I, if you keep this kind of baby. I was wrong." I sat down and continued. "We've been watching videos and researching. I think, given their disadvantages and achievements, people with Down syndrome are more likely to make a difference in the world than the average person. They can and do have meaningful lives."

Erica had searched out and seen many of the same videos we had. "I couldn't work yesterday. I watched videos all day," she told us. Her eyes were puffy, and she had clearly been crying as much as we had, maybe more. "Did you see the video of little Maddox? She beat some incredible odds. She's amazing."

Hearing Erica say that was like music to our ears. We were elated.

"This is our daughter," she stressed.

"We made her," I was surprised to hear Liz say. Then, as abruptly as she had interjected herself into the conversation, she became quiet again.

"We can live with Down syndrome," Erica said, looking at Liz.

But Liz shook her head and muttered, her lower lip trembling, "I don't know about that."

We waited a little longer than usual, but eventually a woman in a brown pinstriped suit came into the waiting room. "Andréa Ott?" she called out.

We all got up and introduced ourselves to her. Her name was Sarah Friedman, Dr. Spencer's genetic counselor. She was a tall, thin, and mousy gal in her early thirties. Her frizzy brown hair was pulled back in a loose ponytail. She led us to her tiny white office that was crammed with a tall bookcase in the corner and a large desk that took up half the room. There were two cramped chairs facing the desk. "Let me get more chairs," Ms. Friedman said, and went to fetch them.

Not knowing how she was going to fit extra chairs in, I offered to stand, but she insisted on finding more. She came back in a minute with two more chairs. Somehow, the four of us managed to maneuver them into the squished space, and soon we were all sitting down. This preliminary delay with the chairs had made us feel even tenser than before.

It was a strange, impersonal meeting. Ms. Friedman began by educating us on Trisomy 21—Down syndrome—chromosomes. She produced charts and illustrations of chromosomes, and then shifted the subject to genetics. "We still do not know what causes Trisomy 21. Down syndrome is spontaneous," she informed us.

I was stunned. "Even with all the advances humans have made? I mean Down syndrome has been around forever. We've found cures for all kinds of diseases. We've sent a man to walk on the moon. We can even clone human beings, but they still don't know how Trisomy is caused? You're kidding me!"

It's because nobody cares!

The first twenty minutes of this meeting had been all about genetic codes, markers, and medical chromosomal mumbo jumbo, but the rest of the meeting took an entirely different and not-so-nice direction.

"Well, from what we know, it typically points to a bad egg from the mother," was her dry proclamation. Thank God, Andréa and I already knew this. We'd found it out from our research the day before.

Apparently, so had Liz and Erica.

"We read that too," Erica said, nodding and looking straight at Andréa.

Ms. Friedman began grilling Andréa over her health, the health of her family, and her medical history. Liz and Erica were paying very close attention.

"Yeah, we were wondering that too," one or the other of them interjected from time to time. I didn't get the feeling that Liz and Erica were wondering these things for the sake of medical research.

Do they think Andréa and I misled them? They think it's her fault? Don't they remember that their own doctor gave Andréa a clean bill of health? I started to feel defensive and protective. I moved my chair up to block Andréa, and I put my hand in her lap, as if I were letting them know I was going to protect her.

Neither Andréa nor I had expected this grilling and finger pointing. Naïvely, we'd thought we were there to learn what it meant for a child to have Down syndrome and, most important, to learn how to deal with it. But it didn't appear that we were going anywhere near those topics.

Ms. Friedman moved on to Shawn and Rod's history. Liz and Erica had called them the night before, and the four of them had speculated about the reasons for the baby's Down syndrome. Ms. Friedman did not spend much time on the two men. It was a perfunctory question-and-answer session, nowhere near as probing as what Andréa had just gone through.

"Both Shawn and Rod have no history...are very healthy," Liz went on. "No problems, no problems at all."

Liz and Erica shook their heads as they answered Ms. Friedman's questions. They made Shawn and Rod sound like textbook perfections of the male body.

I was grateful when Liz changed the direction of the conversation and asked, "I just really want to know what all this means."

Finally, this is what we came here for! Now we'll get some answers.

But to my surprise, Ms. Friedman had none. Other than technical data, statistics, and who to blame, she had no idea what life was like raising a child with Down syndrome. She did know about the medical problems a Down syndrome child was predisposed to. "The baby could have a serious heart defect," she told us.

That wasn't news to us. Dr. Spencer had noted fluid around the baby's heart in the scan. We had talked about it earlier in the waiting room.

"But it's so common in Down syndrome that it's easily fixed with surgery," Erica had said as she described a video she had seen.

We let Ms. Friedman continue. "It could have autism. It could have gastrointestinal problems. No one knows how severely each child will be affected." Her list of all the things that could go wrong was endless. She was really into negatives.

Liz and Erica had many questions. Both Erica and I asked what daily life was like for the parent of a child with Down syndrome, while Liz seemed to want more of the technical what-ifs she was hearing from Ms. Friedman. After the raking over the coals that she had just gotten, Andréa was quiet.

In all honesty, while Ms. Friedman may have been an expert in chromosomes, she had absolutely no idea how to answer most of our real-life questions, at least for Andréa and me.

Andréa and I squeezed each other's hands many times during the meeting, as if to tell each other, *this is bullshit.* We knew from our research that there were also positives, and that many of these negatives were purely hypothetical. We were hoping that all the bad news wasn't affecting Liz and Erica's ability to make a well-thought-out decision.

I mentioned to Ms. Friedman Andréa's discovery of the link between anovulatory cycles before conception and bad eggs. "I wonder if we can indirectly thank the IUD for causing the baby's condition," I said.

"Interesting." Ms. Friedman thought about it. "I'm not sure. I'll find out whether anything has been documented," she said.

The meeting seemed to be coming to an end. We asked Ms. Friedman for a copy of the test results. Before she gave them to us, she wanted to look them over.

Making Matters Worse

Ms. Friedman started to read the report aloud to us. Apparently, this was the first time she had actually read the report herself. She stopped as she read two words that Dr. Spencer had written down: "cystic hygroma." Her flat tone and unexcited attitude changed.

She now had an opinion: "This baby will likely decline on its own."

Andréa and I already knew about cystic hygromas from our research into thick nuchal folds. There was a discussion forum online about a little girl with Down syndrome. At six months' gestation, her thick nuchal fold turned into a cystic hygroma. She passed away in her mother's womb. It's a deadly condition in which fluid builds up in the baby's body and basically drowns it.

This was the first and only time we had heard Peanut had this. It felt odd to me that Dr. Spencer didn't mention it before. He wasn't exactly shy about delivering bad news. Why didn't he mention it when he called with the results? Yet, here he'd written it in the official report. I was immediately suspicious.

"This baby will likely be stillborn," Ms. Friedman repeated to us. "These babies rarely make it to birth. It might pass away soon anyway." She excused herself and left the room for a few moments. When she came back, she said, "Dr. Spencer is not in today, but I talked to his partner, Dr. Lee, and she wanted me to reiterate to you that this baby is not likely to survive." She paused, as if she were thinking how to say something. "Dr. Lee also wanted me to tell you that the staff at this office performs terminations, if you want to schedule one."

This news, while suspicious, was still shocking. As if Down syndrome weren't bad enough, here they were telling us the baby had cystic hygroma too, and was unlikely to survive? I shook my head and indicated to Ms. Freidman that we were not going to make rash decisions. Erica nodded and agreed. I didn't care whether Erica and Liz thought we might be stepping on their toes.

With my doubts of this latest nasty diagnosis, I had to push it. "Can we get another ultrasound to confirm the cystic hygroma?" I curtly asked Ms. Friedman. Erica nodded. Andréa let me take the lead as usual, but she had a bewildered look on her face, looking to me for protection. Liz also looked like a deer in the headlights and didn't say a word.

"Of course," Ms. Friedman replied. "Though if we do one now, nothing will have changed, but we can schedule you for a sixteen-week follow-up ultrasound and see where the baby is."

It would be a long three-week wait, but Andréa and I needed to be sure that what Dr. Spencer had written in his report was true.

We scheduled the follow-up ultrasound, the meeting was over, and the four of us made our way down the hall.

Andréa whispered to me as we walked, "From what I read yesterday, thick nuchal translucency measurements in conjunction with Down syndrome don't always become cystic hygromas." We were on the same page.

I nodded, leaned in, and mentioned my concerns about our just now finding out about this, then said, "We can't just take this guy's word for it. We need to find out more ourselves."

We had just walked out the front door and were in the parking lot saying our goodbyes when Dr. Spencer's office manager came running out of the lobby to catch us. She was a short, thin Hispanic woman with her hair slicked back tightly, maybe too tightly, into a ponytail.

"I thought I'd better let you know that if you continue the pregnancy, there may be significant out-of-pocket expenses for tests that your insurance probably will not cover. They're very expensive," she said abruptly in a snotty tone.

If I hadn't been offended before, I absolutely was now. *Why do they want to kill this baby?* My protective nature was about to kick into overdrive.

Just as directly as she approached us, I gave her a snappy reply with an angry look on my face: "We aren't worried about the costs of tests right now." And with that, the four of us parted ways, got into our cars, and left.

Other than the insinuations against Andréa, we felt that Liz and Erica were still committed to Peanut, or at least Erica certainly was. We were relieved they still called the baby their daughter, even though we sensed that they hadn't entirely closed their minds to termination.

"They do love her!" I told Andréa on the way home.

"We're all on the same page," Andréa agreed and smiled.

Unfortunately, we should have read between the lines. In the days to come, it became evident that Liz was struggling much more than we had recognized. We should have known that Liz, always in control, always an utter perfectionist, and worried nonstop about money, would be unable to see a silver lining in this situation.

Either Erica forgot or chose not to give Andréa her January payment again. This time, though, Andréa was upset.

"I understood their not paying me last week, because everyone was upset, but not paying me this week too? Look at everything I've done—everything for them. What's wrong with them? Where are their hearts?" She wasn't making any more excuses.

A couple days later, Ms. Friedman called to tell me that she had, in fact, found clinical studies showing a possible link between anovulation and Down syndrome.

By now, Andréa and I knew that her IUD was the likely cause of her anovulation.

What Were the Odds?

What were the odds? I needed to know. I found myself sitting at our dining room table on my laptop talking to Peanut's ultrasound picture.

I already knew that eighty percent of babies with Down syndrome miscarried in the first three months. I scratched my head and looked down at the baby in the black-and-white photo. *So, Peanut, girl, you beat those odds.*

But what about this cystic hygroma?

My research documented the general consensus: Less than five percent of babies diagnosed with cystic hygroma survived to be born. If they did, they were born with deformities, usually a huge fluid-filled bubble at the back of their necks, often equal in size to their heads, making them look like they had two heads. They seldom lived long.

I frowned and ran my finger across the photo of Peanut. *I'm not giving up on you, little one.* I couldn't get past the nagging feeling both Andréa and I had that Dr. Spencer was wrong.

Over and over again, I read that many babies with Down syndrome almost always had thick NT measurements due to the delay of development of their lymphatic systems. Sometimes, and especially in babies with Down syndrome, once the lymphatic system became fully developed, the fluid resolved itself before twenty-four weeks and in reality never turned into a cystic hygroma at all.

Andréa came in and sat next to me. I told her what I had learned.

She was baffled. "There must be some reason he diagnosed it as a cystic hygroma. Something we're missing?"

There was a bigger black cloud hanging over Peanut—even bigger than cystic hygroma.

The Days that Followed

Andréa and I did not get the answers to our most important questions at the genetic counseling meeting, but I wasn't going to give up.

I called our local Down syndrome organization, the Down Syndrome Connection of the Bay Area (DSC); I explained our diagnosis to the woman on the phone. I was full of questions: Did they have resources about cystic hygroma? Should we get a second opinion? I was put right through to the founder, who ran the organization, and she told me that she would ask their advising doctor, a leading pediatrician whose specialty was Down syndrome.

That night Andréa and I were lying in bed when she felt Peanut move for the first time. It was as if she were telling Andréa, "I'm here, I'm fighting." It was bittersweet. I was proud of this little fighter.

Andréa texted Erica and got an unenthusiastic, "That's nice." Erica's short, uninterested reply worried Andréa and me.

A few days later, the founder of the DSC called me back with interesting news relayed from their specialist: "At thirteen weeks, it's difficult to diagnose a fetus that has Down syndrome with cystic hygroma. It's too soon."

Well, that's what we thought, but the report clearly stated the baby has cystic hygroma.

As soon as we heard that news confirming our suspicions, we wanted to share it with Erica. I texted her right away and told her what I'd learned from the specialist. I got his telephone number from the DSC and urged her to set up an appointment for all of us.

Erica did not respond. *Uh-oh!*

The next day I finally received a text from her: "Liz and I have an appointment next Friday with another geneticist privately. We are talking over our case and possible prognosis."

The word *privately* spoke volumes to me. I debated whether or not to tell Andréa about it.

"Not Sarah Friedman? I hope this person isn't biased," I texted back. I understood their desire not to involve us, but this was a concern.

"No, Sarah actually referred us to him. He can just provide more data. He's an outside source who is not involved with our case at all, and he can give us an unbiased opinion," Erica replied.

It was all very matter-of-fact. My concern was mounting.

They want more data? Why would they see another geneticist? Why not see a doctor who specializes in Down syndrome? Someone who actually knows about this disability?

This was the first obvious sign of dissension between them and us. I decided not to tell Andréa.

Over the next week, Andréa came across a study in a behavioral neuroscience magazine authored by a Cornell University professor, Doctor Barbara Strupp, that explored the effects on mice with simulated Down syndrome who were given a dietary supplement called choline. It was discovered that the mice had "dramatic reduction in dysfunction" caused by the simulated Down syndrome. This was the kind of information that we had hoped to find out from the genetic counselor, but hadn't.

So off we went to the vitamin store to stock up on choline, and Andréa began taking it that very day.

I texted Erica and told her about choline. Her replies were becoming one-liners: "That makes sense, since it is brain food."

I kept on urging her: "We need to just wait and see what happens at the ultrasound." It was still a long ten days away.

Over the next few days, Erica and I texted each other often, and during this time, it felt like I was communicating with two different people. Sometimes she gave me the impression she wanted to keep the baby and was going to fight for her, but then in the very next text, she would tell me all the reasons she was hesitant. She was clearly torn.

When I repeated to her what the DSC specialist had told us, she replied, "We hope the cystic hygroma gets better, but we have to be realistic. I am a hundred percent behind the baby, but..." The "but..." went on and on about all the possible horrible things that could go wrong.

I wondered what was going on in their minds. Very soon, the texts started to reveal how Liz and Erica were leaning.

"Liz is having a hard time dealing with this. This weekend she had a mini breakdown." Erica also added, "Liz's mom is not being supportive and putting pressure on Liz." This was the first time we knew about this other very difficult aspect that Liz was dealing with. She could not stand up to her mom, who was an even greater perfectionist than Liz was herself.

"Liz can give herself permission to be a better woman," I texted back to Erica. I went on to explain about my mother and how I knew she would have felt the same as Liz's. I hoped Erica would repeat my story to Liz. "I also know that at the end of the day, this child would probably have been my mother's favorite grandchild."

Erica agreed and seemed to feel better for the moment, but her respite was short-lived. "This is by far the hardest thing I have ever had to deal with, besides my mom dying," she texted me. My heart ached for Erica, but there was a new person involved now, one I had to protect.

The next morning, I was driving home from picking up paint at the hardware store when I got a text from Erica's number. From the tone, I felt like it was written by Liz, not Erica.

"We want you to know we aren't a hundred percent sure we aren't going to terminate. It is a very personal decision, and ours alone to make, and not one we take lightly, but there are a lot of factors to consider. We haven't made a decision yet. This is a very difficult choice! I hope you respect that. Liz is really struggling with all of this."

Whoa! Wait, they think it's their personal decision, and theirs alone, to terminate Andréa's biological child? I was stunned. I couldn't understand how they could swat away Andréa's and my feelings about this like a fly on the wall. I was angry. No one was going to stop this baby girl from fighting for her life. No one had a crystal ball that could reveal the truth about all the horrible things everyone was predicting, but all of them sure were acting like they had.

There were too many people deciding whether she was going to live or die, and I realized she herself did not have a say. At that point, as sad as I was for Liz and Erica, I was going to ensure that Peanut had a voice in this.

I decided not to hide this last text from Andréa. I got home from my errands and handed her my cell phone so she could read them all.

"It's done. It's over for them. They don't deserve her," she said without a second thought.

"Panda, they're going through a lot. Let's ask to meet them for dinner and talk to them. Let's see how they really feel," I insisted.

"It's so sad that we have to save this baby from her own intended mothers." Andréa looked disgusted.

I knew that from that moment on, it would be hard if not impossible for Liz and Erica to recover in Andréa's eyes. I almost felt that fate had given them a test, and they had failed. At this point, I was sure we would be keeping the baby ourselves. That day, the ten months of all our efforts for Liz and Erica ended. Even though I felt tremendous guilt and sorrow for them, I knew what we had to do. We had to save this baby. I couldn't look back.

Still, I didn't want to hurt them or lash out. I had Andréa, who had turned into a mama bear, but I was also sympathetic to the crushed dreams of Liz and Erica on the other side. While I couldn't understand that they felt we had no choice, I did understand where Liz was coming from; I had just recently been there. But regardless, Andréa did not want to give her disabled cub to people she now deemed unworthy. I had to let Liz and Erica go.

Peanut *did* have mothers who loved her and believed in her, even if no one else would. We were her real moms.

For finality, I felt we needed to hear certainty from Liz and Erica's own mouths. "I think we have to give them one last chance, Panda. We need to hear them say they don't want her before we do this." She agreed, but mama bear was baring her sharp teeth.

We let a few days go by. Eventually I had to text Erica. I was blunt: "We're not feeling that you are on board anymore."

Erica replied to my text, "We have to be realistic. Why do you guys feel we're not on board?"

It was a sensitive subject. Should I tell her: "Because your mama bear doesn't seem to exist?" Should I tell her: "A mama bear wouldn't say, 'Gee, I hope the cystic hygroma gets better, but...?'"

I couldn't throw that at them now. I still didn't know what to say, so I skirted the question and came up with something else. It wasn't what we were feeling so passionate about, but it was still an issue that had to be addressed, and this was as good an opportunity as any to get it over with. I texted, "It seems like you might be bowing out, because you guys didn't pay Andréa for January after we found out the baby has DS."

A few minutes passed; then I received a response from Erica. "We forgot," she apologized. "I will put it in the mail."

At this point, Andréa and I could have cared less about the money; but there was the principle. It was wrong. But Erica got around answering the question directly. We didn't care whether they ever caught up. We didn't care whether we ever received another dime from them. But we did care about Peanut. We cared about her deeply. We weren't about to kill her because *they* were afraid.

But Erica again reiterated by text "terminating is a personal matter."

I felt like she was telling me to butt out, and I was angry. *Well, no, dear, terminating is actually not your decision at all.* I bit my tongue, but had wild thoughts running through my head that I would have liked to unload.

I felt I should consider the legal aspect of this. Liz and Erica had said more than once that termination was their choice alone, and that alarmed Andréa and me. *Are they thinking they have the legal right to make that decision? How can they? That makes no sense.*

Andréa found the surrogacy agreement in our file cabinet. About halfway through, we realized there was, in fact, a clause in our contract that stated "If for medical reasons Intended Parents choose to terminate, surrogate agrees to abide by their wishes," meaning that we had agreed to terminate the baby if Liz and Erica wanted us to. We were horrified and scared.

After I calmed myself down, I texted Erica, letting her know that if they didn't want to keep the baby, it was okay. "This needs to be said,"

I wrote her. "Andréa and I will release you from all your liabilities the second you tell us you do not want the baby."

"Thank you; I appreciate your saying that," she replied.

I hoped this would stop her from declaring that terminating the baby was their decision, and their decision alone. I was offering them the chance to bow out gracefully.

CHAPTER 12

No Dinner at All

January 25, 2013

I HOPED LIZ AND ERICA WOULD HAVE A HEART-TO-heart talk with us, and that they would stop bouncing around "termination" and "our choice"—meaning "not yours"—statements. You would have had to be an idiot not to see the writing on the wall, and I knew there was no way in hell Andréa would forgive them and hand the baby over at this point.

"They have to tell us themselves they don't want her," I told Andréa again. "We need to meet."

We arranged to meet Liz and Erica for dinner after their appointment with their private geneticist. Andréa and I already had pretty good idea where this meeting was likely to go.

We met at Mexico Lindo, a restaurant in Pleasanton, midway between their house and ours. Mexico Lindo had one very large room, like a warehouse with a high, open ceiling. There were a few Mexican decorations around the place—a huge Mexican sun and a bunch of sombreros hung on the walls—but our chief impression was that the place was just crowded and loud. A quieter place might have been better for our candid talk.

Andréa and I arrived early in our usual fashion and had to wait for at least half an hour before Liz and Erica walked in. They quickly spotted us in the crowded dining room. As we hugged and sat down, they apologized for being so late. Their little dog had eaten a bag of "edibles," as they put it, that belonged to a houseguest. The dog had overdosed on them.

"Your dog OD'd on bad fruit?" I asked, incredulously thinking that they were talking about edible fruit bouquets.

"No, she ate a bag of edibles," Erica repeated, as if she were being perfectly clear.

I was completely mystified.

Andréa clarified: "Pot, babe. She ate a bag of edible pot." With a crooked smile, she squeezed my hand tightly under the table.

Holy shit! What if that had been the baby!

At least it helped us get off to a cordial start. We ordered our food.

Erica sat across from me, while Liz sat across from Andréa. Erica handed Andréa an envelope, her belated January payment. Andréa looked over at me as if asking whether she should accept it. I whispered quietly in her ear, "Yes, of course you should. They should have given it to you on the first, not the twenty-fifth."

From the look of Erica's puffy red eyes, she had clearly been crying a lot. Liz appeared numb, worn down. Her chin was shaking, as if she were on the verge of a nervous breakdown, and for the first part of the evening, she was barely able to maintain composure. I felt very sorry for her.

We shared annoying small talk, pretending there wasn't any eight-hundred-pound gorilla lurking invisibly at the table with us. It took a while before Erica could bring herself to acknowledge its presence: She revealed that their private geneticist had confirmed their worst fears. "All these other terrible things could also be wrong with the baby," she told us. "We would be getting a grab-bag full of horrific unknowns. The baby could be blind…could be a vegetable…it could have a grotesque deformity behind its neck," she went on. "That is, if it lives." Erica wasn't calling the baby "Peanut" anymore.

I squeezed Andréa's hand. I must admit that she and I felt a bit of relief. We had already made this decision for them and were glad that they seemed to be on the same page.

While Liz was talking to Andréa, Erica told me under her breath, "I have to choose either my wife or my daughter." Erica was still struggling and my heart ached for her. I knew she wanted to keep the baby.

I told Erica what she already knew. "Andréa and I are prepared to keep her. You don't need to worry. Everything will be okay." But Liz was listening in now, and that was when the evening started to take a nasty turn.

Once again, I brought up what the DSC specialist had told us about cystic hygromas in babies with Down syndrome.

Andréa also chimed in: "According to the DSC specialist, it's much too early for Dr. Spencer to diagnose cystic hygroma." She was making sure they heard her one last time.

"The geneticist we saw today read Dr. Spencer's report himself, and he is very knowledgeable about the complications of cystic hygromas," Liz interjected defensively.

It was no use; Liz and Erica wanted to believe and focus only on the negatives. Eventually I excused myself to use the bathroom. To my surprise, I turned around and noticed Liz following me.

Inside the restroom, she confronted me accusingly. "How could you possibly support keeping this baby? You didn't even want a baby." She was shaking badly. "It will never amount to anything," she said hopelessly.

I felt sorry for her.

"Liz, what is it to you? What does it matter? It's Andréa's biological child." I was disappointed in her. Why couldn't she see this? Why was she holding on so adamantly? She wasn't going to be responsible for this child. We had assured her of that.

I tried to make her see that she was being unreasonable. "You won't have to pay us anymore for the surrogacy. You won't have to have a termination on your conscience. Everything will be okay."

She was beyond logic and couldn't hear me. "I can't live with myself if you keep this baby," she said angrily, half in tears, and then she started rambling on about all the bad things the baby would likely turn out to have.

I was at a loss and hurting over her pain. "I'm so sorry, I'm so sorry," was all I could get in between her incoherent words.

I knew I needed to get out of the bathroom. I opened the door and Liz darted out in front of me.

"I'm going to talk to Andréa about this," she declared vehemently, and headed for our table.

Not wanting her to attack Andréa, I followed right at her heels. She stopped dead in her tracks, turned on me, and, pointing her finger at my face, said, "You are facing a lawsuit if you do not terminate." Then she turned back around and continued toward the table.

We both made it there at the same time. I didn't give Liz the opportunity to confront Andréa.

"Get your things. We're leaving." Our dinner had just arrived and we hadn't even begun to eat.

"Sit back down. I want to talk to you," Liz said imperiously. She still looked shaken, but was more composed than she had been just a brief second ago.

"No, I'm so sorry, but no." Laying my palm flat on the table, I looked straight at her and then helped Andréa stand up. Andréa took out her wallet, and Erica, who looked stunned, waved her hand.

"We have this," Erica said.

Andréa and I walked out. From that moment on, it was me, Andréa, and the baby against the world.

That was the last time we ever saw Liz and Erica.

Can They Sue Us;
Can They Make Us Terminate?

We were really worried. As if Andréa didn't have enough on her plate with everything that was going on, along with her still-hard-hitting morning sickness, now we had to worry about a possible lawsuit. Could a judge force us to terminate?

Andréa's cousin Nikki was an attorney. We asked for her help and sent her a copy of our surrogacy agreement. It took her a few days to evaluate, but she called at last to give us her opinion.

She started talking in legal terms and jargon until I asked, "Can they force Andréa to terminate her own biological child?" That was the nightmare question hanging over us.

"They could try," Nikki answered. "They could try to sue you for breach of contract, but their own contract was breached when you used fresh sperm instead of frozen and when they didn't pay you as they'd legally agreed to." She paused. "In the end, no court would ever force you to terminate your own child," she told us. "The clause shouldn't have been in here. It's unconscionable and unenforceable."

Andréa and I sighed with relief as Nikki continued talking.

She was frank with us: "Look, they can find an attorney who will take their money and take their case. So if they want to try to sue you, they can. They won't win, but they can try. No judge would want to come near this thing with a ten-foot pole," she added.

And with that, we hung up, still feeling nervous, but our burden of fear was not quite as heavy. A court battle wasn't what we needed right now.

And Then There Were Three
January 27, 2013

After talking with Andréa's cousin, we decided we needed to formally dissolve our agreement with Liz and Erica. Andréa typed up a letter of dissolution, and we sent it by certified mail.

I felt terrible. I hated how this was playing out.

Obviously, Liz could not handle raising a child with Down syndrome, and someone had to release her from her guilt and pain. Like the nine out of ten parents who aborted a baby diagnosed with the condition, Liz knew what she could and could not manage. No one could judge her for that. I might never have seen inside my own heart without the strength of my love for Andréa and her wise and subtle ways. I'm positive I would have made the same decision as Liz.

Liz was coming across as the bad guy, and I felt really terrible about that, but I was a champion for a new person—Peanut. I could not be so concerned with Liz or Erica. They had to take care of each other now. For Andréa and me now, it had to be about this baby girl who hadn't asked to be created, certainly wasn't asking to be terminated, and was fighting for her life at this very moment.

But Andréa and I had removed the biggest threat to her life.

We didn't want our letter to surprise Erica. Andréa texted her and asked her to call. We were sitting on our bed watching TV when she did. Andréa turned off the TV and put her phone on speaker mode.

"We don't want to shock you," Andréa told Erica gently. She went on to explain that there needed to be a formal dissolution, and we were sending them a letter spelling it out.

"It's the Down syndrome," Erica admitted. "Liz just cannot handle a baby with Down syndrome. You have to understand what a perfectionist Liz is."

This was hardly news to us, though maybe we couldn't understand what a burden it was for her. Erica added that Liz's parents' disapproval was a determining factor too. It was all too much for Liz to bear.

Even though Andréa had the phone on speaker, I stayed out of it and left the room. She and Erica needed to have this final private conversation. I had just walked back into the bedroom when I heard Erica say, "I had to make my choice. It was too much for Liz, and I had to let her off the hook. I cannot force this on her. If I do, she'll either leave me or she will resent me." Erica hesitated. "And I hope I don't come to resent her instead."

Andréa apologized for our leaving so abruptly from dinner. "Keston is protective of me, and when Liz threatened to sue us, Keston felt—"

Erica interrupted and quickly put out that fire. "Liz was just upset and emotional. There will be no lawsuit." She must have felt that she still had to explain. "Liz told me she doesn't want you to have the baby because she'll have to look at herself in the mirror and see what a shallow person she is. I mean, no one is likely to think that, but she will. Knowing the baby is out there is going to distress her always."

I whispered to Andréa to let Erica know we were okay with her.

"Erica, we know you didn't want this. If you want to be in the baby's life, if you want to be Auntie Erica, you're always welcome. There's an open door for you." Andréa's loving nature spilled over toward Erica.

"Thank you, I appreciate that," Erica responded a little shakily, and with that, the conversation ended. Andréa hung up.

It was over. Andréa and I were officially Peanut's mamas. We didn't know at the time, but we'd always been her mamas. She would have had it no other way.

If we'd thought it was going to be smooth sailing from thereon out, we were out of our minds! We were about to find out that I wasn't the only one with a monster hiding in the mirror.

Uncles or Idiots?
January 29, 2013

I have to give Erica credit; over the next few weeks, she checked in on the baby before and after every appointment. I told her, "This baby is going to change the world, Erica. She's going to make a difference." My heart was sure.

"I hope you're right," Erica replied, less convinced.

One day, Erica texted me that Shawn and Rod still wanted to be uncles, and asked us to contact them.

Andréa and I were a little mystified.

Throughout the insemination process, the guys had been mostly polite, but not exactly gracious or friendly to us. However, perhaps their hearts had changed too.

"Of course they can still be uncles," I responded. Andréa and I both agreed. We would send them Facebook friend requests and write an email to Shawn and Rod right away.

That night, I emailed them and told them we absolutely wanted to keep them as uncles, adding, "We need all the help, love, and support we can get...the more people who love this baby, the better!" We told them that we would keep them in the loop as to how the baby was doing.

Most important, we encouraged them to be involved and let them know the door was open.

Very strangely, it seemed to us, they did not reply. It was as if we had told a bad joke and were waiting for laughter. Instead, all we heard was crickets.

A few days after I sent the email, Erica called me. She said, "Shawn and Rod are freaking out. They say you want money. They say they 'can't afford no baby.' They just did their taxes and make less than fifty thousand dollars a year between them."

"What? We didn't ask them for any financial support. What's going on with them?" I was completely taken aback.

"I don't know. That's just what they said," Erica replied.

"Well, I can send you my email." I was angry and wanted to prove my innocence.

"No need."

We got off the phone. I was totally perplexed and offended.

I told Andréa about my conversation with Erica, and I began ranting. "What weirdos! What on earth were these idiots thinking? Besides, didn't they just have their own surrogate and were trying to make a baby with her?"

We stuck this bewildering question on the back burner and tried to forget about it. We hoped Shawn and Rod would simply fade out of the picture. There were more important things to deal with.

We didn't even know whether Peanut was still alive.

CHAPTER 13

Our Warrior from Heaven

January 30, 2013

ANDRÉA WANTED THE BABY TO HAVE AN IDENTITY. She wanted to give her a name. We weren't sure of the fate of this child, but she'd already proven to be such a little fighter, beating the odds left and right.

We decided to name her Delaney, which means "descendant of warriors," and gave her the middle name Skye, which means "heaven," as she was our warrior from heaven. You'll soon see why.

By now, I had played the little red teddy bear song to her so many times that the mechanism no longer worked and the bear no longer sang. So I started singing the song to Delaney every day, but now I changed the words: "Let me call you sweetheart / I'm in love with Delaney Skye / Let me hear you whisper / that you love Mommy O too."

Since I am the cool, fun mom, the kids call me "Mommy-O."

I continued to sing to Andréa's belly every day.

Our love for little Delaney was immense. We couldn't help but admire her. She had already had such a big impact on our lives. She had made such a difference in me. We were so proud of her already, and she wasn't even here yet!

Big Brother, Big Sister!

Andréa and I put a lot of thought into how Jared and Julianna would be affected by having a sibling with Down syndrome. According to our reading, siblings of children with Down syndrome tend to grow up to be unusually compassionate people. Often they become advocates, therapists, and doctors. We met some people at the DSC who provided us with useful resources.

One woman had an interesting story to tell about how close her sons were. Her older son grew up to be a doctor and a strong advocate for his little brother, who had Down syndrome. As a teenager, when he met a girl he liked, he would bring her home without telling her anything about his little brother's disability beforehand. He did it on purpose. How she reacted told him all he needed to know about her.

How weird this situation must have been for Jared and Julianna. They went from being "cousins of sorts" to "Well, now she's going to be your little sister, and not only is she your sister, but she has something called Down syndrome. She will be different."

We sat them down at the dinner table one night and let the kids know we had something to tell them. "We're keeping the baby we were making for Liz and Erica," I said, fully expecting them to be very confused about it.

"But this isn't our baby." Jared looked at me wide-eyed, repeating what I had been telling him for months, as his mother got bigger.

"We were making the baby for Liz and Erica, but they don't want her anymore. So since she's your mom's and your blood, we want her. We love her," I told them. *How in the world can I explain to them what "biological mother" means?* I tried to find terms they could understand. "She really is your sister. We were just going to let Liz and Erica raise her," was the best I could do. "We're naming her Delaney, and we're keeping her."

"Why don't Liz and Erica want her?" Jared asked.

Oh, man, this is tough!

Andréa and I looked at each other, trying to find words of wisdom. I'm not sure those words ever came, but we tried.

"Because she might be sick, and she has something called Down syndrome," Andréa said.

And I added, "It will make her different. She won't learn things as fast as other kids. Some people might be mean to her. It's too scary for Liz and Erica."

We knew we couldn't really explain things that they would comprehend. They would have to understand in time.

I decided to lighten the conversation up. "Delaney might have a hard time talking, so we're all going to learn sign language to help her."

Andréa and I wanted Delaney to have the same opportunities as some of the babies in the videos we had seen. She was going to have a head start in life. We would help her as a family, as a team.

That night, we started going over sign words at the dinner table, "So you guys can teach Delaney." They understood that; that was fun!

Congratulations! You're Grandparents!
January 31, 2013

You just couldn't have asked for better grandparents than Andréa's parents and their new spouses, Boppi's partner Robin, whom the kids called "Grams," and Tutu's husband Scott, who was "Grandpa." All four were such an integral part of Jared and Julianna's lives, and it never dawned on us that they would feel any differently about Delaney.

We were cautious, yet naïve. We had finally sold them on the idea of Andréa's being a surrogate, but now we had to tell them that we would be keeping the baby. And, by the way, they would be grandparents to a child with Down syndrome.

This baby needs her grandparents, all four of them, to be her champions too. And so do Andréa and I.

Andréa would have been more than happy never to tell her parents that we were keeping the baby, but it had to be done. Boppi's caring reaction when Andréa had told him about the baby's condition made her feel a little less stressed about telling him. But Tutu was a different story. Telling Tutu filled Andréa with dread.

Everyday I asked her, "Have you told your parents yet?"

And everyday she would tell me, "No, not yet."

After a few days of this, it became frustrating. "Why the hell not? They're a huge part of our kids' lives."

But Andréa ignored my frustration and continued to brush me off.

I refused to let the matter drop and kept on grilling her. Finally, she gave me a quick answer: "Because I always let them down, especially my mom. I don't think I can take it if they don't approve."

"Your dad supports you in everything you do," I argued with her. "People are going to start to know, so how do you think your mom and dad will feel if they're the last to find out?"

I finally got through to Andréa with that, only she still refused to call them. Instead, she decided to write them an email. "I don't want them to cut me off, ask questions, and talk over me," she explained. "This way they have to read and hear everything I say before they push their own opinions onto me."

Even knowing how Andréa dealt with confrontation, I thought this was a fraidy-cat way out of it. However, it was the best she could do. She wrote both of them the same, somewhat formal email:

Boppi and Mom,

I really need your help and support more than ever before. Liz and Erica have decided they cannot move forward with the pregnancy. I am really hurt and sad. I don't understand how two people could want a baby so much and then change their mind just because she is not the "perfect" baby they dreamed of. I can't go along with them and agree that she does not deserve to live because she is different. This baby was *wanted* and made with *love*. I just cannot terminate this little girl who was brought into this world with the best intentions and obviously is here for a reason.

There is a chance that she won't make it, but there is also a chance that she will. She is a strong little one. She's already surpassed the doctors' expectations, and it's clear she is fighting for her life. She wants to be here, and I don't have any doubts that she will make it. We feel she is a special gift and will make a wonderful addition to our family.

I know that you may have mixed emotions and a lot of questions as you are hearing this. We had mixed emotions too—not about the Down syndrome, but about having a *baby*. This is not at all what we intended, but like Keston says, "Sometimes you don't get what you want; you get what you need."

I really need your support through this very emotional time and certainly understand that at first you might not know what to say. Please be considerate and understand that we have made our choice to let her fight. We recognize that she will give not only us, but all of our family and friends such a unique opportunity that we otherwise might not have had. Once we talked to other families through the Down Syndrome Connection in Danville who have children with Down syndrome, we realized right away that there are not any regrets and only love and pride in their children. Children with Down syndrome are more like "typical" kids than one might first think. She will be able to do many of the same things (in her own time) and live a happy life.

To help you understand what this means for our family, I hope you will take some time to research Down syndrome. The more educated we are, the better life we will be able to provide her. To help get you started, please watch these videos and read the "Grandparent Packet."

We are really looking forward—and hope you will too—to meeting Delaney Skye, which loosely translates to "warrior from heaven."

Love,
Andréa

Boppi called later that night. Andréa let the phone go to voicemail.

"Chicken!" I joked with her to make light of her stress. "You have to call him back." And she did. Boppi had had a change of heart—a dark change of heart.

"I think you should terminate," were the first words out of his mouth. This cold, blunt statement coming from the man she trusted most was a low blow for Andréa.

Andréa's response was quick, and she was mad: "I didn't ask you for your opinion or approval. I only ask that you accept this baby as your grandchild."

"This is going to be a hard life. She could have other things wrong with her. What if she's blind? Do you want that to happen to her?" His voice was raised, and it rattled with concern.

Boppi's boss had a child with Down syndrome who was legally blind. Like my own fears due to my experience, or lack thereof, this was all that Boppi knew about Down syndrome. He was scared for us.

Andréa was on the defensive now. "The baby isn't going to be blind, but if she is, we'll deal with it."

"Well, I don't think it would be good for Jared. This baby is going to take attention away from him. He's going to grow up to be a jerk, or even violent like his father." Boppi was starting to sound desperate. We thought it was very odd that he mentioned only Jared and said nothing about Julianna. I felt as if I should leave the room and let them have this conversation, but with her free hand, Andréa held on to mine tightly, like a security blanket. She started to cry as she spoke.

"If you can't support me, you will lose me," she told him. I was shocked to hear her speak to her dad this way. "I'm only asking that you accept this baby. She's your blood, Boppi." Andréa's lip was trembling. "I want you to be as good a grandpa for her as you are for Jared and Julianna."

The two stubborn stallions held their ground. Boppi wouldn't budge. "It's going to be expensive. How are you going to afford the medical bills?" His tone was sharp.

"Disabled children qualify for Medi-Cal, Boppi." Andréa explained to him the different state programs the baby would be eligible for: Medi-Cal, occupational, physical, and speech therapies, et cetera.

On the other end of the phone Boppi was not convinced and didn't seem to listen to what Andréa was telling him. Even though she had already answered his questions about medical insurance, he kept going on about the medical costs of having a disabled baby as if he thought Andréa were lying to him.

It was clear that nothing she said was going to make Boppi change his mind right now, but before he got off the phone, he did tell her, very unconvincingly, "Of course I will support you." And without saying much else, he hung up.

We sat there and looked at each other in distress and bewilderment. "If Jared ever found out we'd terminated his little sister because we thought he'd be a jerk, he'd never forgive us," I said to Andréa. "He's a sensitive little boy. Boppi doesn't know him very well if that's what he thinks about him."

"I agree," Andréa answered, but was too hurt to say much more.

"How did he go from 'it's too late to terminate' when we originally found out the baby might have Down syndrome to 'now you should terminate'?" I couldn't process that.

"Robin must have changed his mind," Andréa sighed.

Being a daddy's girl, she hadn't expected this kind of reaction from Boppi. She was deeply hurt.

Andréa was only twelve when her parents divorced. And she didn't take it well. She resented Boppi and blamed him for the breakup of their family—for not having been around, for working too much during the week, and for playing soccer on the weekends—and she had taken it out on him.

As she grew up, she came to realize there was more to the end of her parents' marriage than she had ever understood. She saw that Boppi realized his mistakes and had suffered greatly. "He loved my mom and he lost her. He didn't want to lose me," she would tell me.

In her late teens, after her mother remarried, she spent more and more time with her father.

"I've never met anyone who doesn't have great respect for my dad," she had told me when I first met her. Somewhere along the line, Boppi became Andréa's confidant and perhaps even her best friend. Much as I had turned to my mother, Andréa went to Boppi when she needed advice.

Because of how close they were today, it was hard for Andréa to have Boppi not support her decision; however, with a tender wisdom beyond her years, Andréa worked through her hurt. She knew Boppi was scared for her and the children. "He needs time. I know it's because he loves us. He's worried about what this might mean for me and the kids." Andréa understood his fear, but she wasn't afraid to tell him he was wrong if she had to.

It was weeks before Tutu answered, and when she did, it was via email. While her response wasn't nearly as surprising as Boppi's, it was plain that she thought this was a bad idea. "You will always have my love, but I do not support this decision. You both have big hearts, and that is all you are thinking with right now," she wrote.

Like Boppi, she was concerned about Jared and Julianna, the attention they would miss out on, and how cruel other children might be when they found out about their little sister. She was also worried about how we were going to afford a special-needs child. She suggested we put the baby up for adoption. She was short and to the point, but she was more loving in her tone than Andréa had expected.

"At least she doesn't say I should terminate." Andréa was glad of that.

From both their responses, we were pretty sure neither of her parents had taken the time to watch the videos or read the information Andréa had sent them. It was another hard blow for her, but not nearly enough to make her change her mind.

Andréa and I would never waver.

How Do We Explain...
We Accidently Got Pregnant?
February 3, 2013

One of the first things we learned while visiting the Down syndrome advocacy websites was that we would have to lead by example. We should be direct, honest, and proud.

When Andréa became pregnant, we knew people would soon start to notice it, so we had announced we were doing the surrogate thing. But now, in a bizarre twist of fate, we were keeping the baby, and she had Down syndrome. Sooner or later, people were going to know and maybe start gossiping, and we needed to head that off.

We took a cue from the experts, the Down syndrome advocates. Many suggested making an announcement. That way it would be out in the open and people would have time to absorb what we were telling them. It would also quash gossip.

Consequently, Andréa spent a day authoring the announcement, and we published the following letter on Facebook, the forum that could reach anyone and everyone.

Dear Family and Friends,

As many of you know, I decided to be a traditional surrogate (my egg and donor sperm) for some family friends. We did genetic testing and are happy to announce that it's a little *girl*! We also found out through the genetic testing that she is positive (99 percent accuracy) for Trisomy 21, more commonly known as Down syndrome.

Many children who are diagnosed with Down syndrome also have other medical issues, and many do not even make it to birth. Understandably, the intended parents were overwhelmed by the unknowns and decided to not move forward with the pregnancy. Lucky for this little girl, Keston and I saw her fighting for her life and could not bear to take that away from her. She is continuing to fight and thrive and surpass all the doctors' expectations. She is a strong little one, and we feel she will make a wonderful addition to our family.

We know that many of you may have mixed emotions and a lot of questions as you are hearing this. We appreciate any and all support and certainly understand that you might not know what to say. You may want to reach out to us via phone, email, or however, but we know it may be hard figuring out what to say to us. Seriously, a simple "congratulations" works just fine. Please understand and be considerate that we have already moved past the emotional turmoil and have moved on to excitement as we eagerly await the arrival of our beautiful baby girl.

We recognize that she will not only give us, but also all of you, such a unique opportunity that we otherwise might not have had. Once we talked to other families who have children with Down syndrome, we realized right away there is never any regret and only love and pride in their child. Children with Down syndrome are more like "typical" kids than one might first think. She will be able to do many of the same things (in her own time) and live a happy life.

We don't want anyone to feel sorry for her or us. We want you to be happy for our family. We would love to know that you are there for us with your love and support. If you were to ask us what you can do to help, we would tell you:

Do not treat our baby or us any differently.

Think before you use the "R" word, laugh, or make fun of someone with a disability.

Help and contribute to society by becoming less afraid and more accepting of those with a disability.

We are really excited to be a part of the Down syndrome community and look forward to kicking adversity and discrimination's butt! We hope you will join us in our fight and help raise awareness.

We really feel lucky to have you all as friends and family, and cannot wait for you to meet Delaney Skye, meaning our "warrior from heaven."

Andréa, Keston, Jared, and Julianna

After reading Andréa's Facebook post, I felt overwhelmed with shame about the person I used to be. Here I was asking our friends and family not to be afraid and to be more accepting of people like Delaney when I myself would have been repulsed. Would people respond at all? Would they ignore this announcement, maybe unfriend us? I would have to be understanding. They couldn't possibly know the great gift and love that I had been given by my muse, by Delaney. Even if they were repulsed (as I would have been only a few months ago), I hoped they wouldn't block or delete us. I knew in my heart of hearts that Delaney had only just begun to teach many beautiful lessons. They would grow too if they just hung on and watched her grow up in our posts.

Knowing how private Liz and Erica are, I also wondered how they might take our announcement. They probably harbored guilt like me, only I looked like a hero in this and they looked cold-hearted, even though Andréa tried to thwart those thoughts by saying nice things about them. I anticipated hearing from them. Andréa didn't agree with me, but I was right. Later that night we were lying in bed, having our usual talk time, when Andréa received a text from Erica. She read it to me, exclamation points and all.

"'I've got to say I am hurt by your Facebook post! I don't feel that you needed to talk about our private arrangement on Facebook! It is out there for everyone to see and I have already had friends call me! Can you please keep that stuff between us?'" Andréa was still reading the first text from Erica to me when another popped up on her cell phone.

"It certainly is still very painful for us, and it didn't seem necessary for you to blast it out to everyone on Facebook! If you could keep that to yourself, I would really appreciate that! I understand you have to explain to close friends and family! Just not everyone! It didn't make us sound very good!"

Andréa was mad. "Fuck them!" I was surprised to hear her curse; she rarely did.

I was calm. "I can kinda see how that might have hurt them," I said. "They're just reacting. You should apologize and tell her you didn't mean to hurt their feelings." I was trying to appease her and help her sympathize with Liz and Erica a little. But her rage against them had simmered too long.

"Apologize? Why should I apologize? I said nice things about them in that announcement so that they *didn't* sound bad, and I'm sorry, now I...," she paused. "They were awful, and we don't have mutual friends. So that's bullshit!"

"I can still see how they might be offended, babe." I tried to make her see their side. "Just apologize for me."

Andréa handed me her phone. "You apologize for me. I'm not going to be sorry for them ever again."

I pretended I was Andréa and texted an apology to Erica.

She accepted it and seemed to feel better, but Andréa was still bitter.

Delaney's Fighting Spirit
February 4, 2013

Even though only a few weeks had passed, it felt like we had been waiting an eternity before the day of our follow-up ultrasound with Dr. Spencer arrived. We might finally get some answers.

We were nervous and I probably drove a little too fast over Kirker Pass to the appointment. We had so many life-and-death questions about our little warrior that might be answered this day

Was Delaney's condition going to be worse? Would Dr. Spencer reconfirm his diagnosis of cystic hygroma? What about the fluid in her chest? Was that nuchal fold behind her neck bigger? We knew it would probably grow worse before it got better, even if it wasn't a cystic hygroma.

Was Delaney even alive anymore? We had felt fluttering in Andréa's stomach, but perhaps that was just gas or hope.

Our tears were already welling as we drove into the parking lot.

My phone vibrated. It was Erica. "Good luck," she wrote. I read it to Andréa. We both smiled and walked into Dr. Spencer's office hand in hand, ready to face whatever was to come.

Earlier in the month, we'd found out that for all his horrid bedside manner, Dr. Spencer was considered one of the best perinatal doctors in the Bay Area. So we decided to keep him. I'm honestly not sure we had much of a choice. But knowing his pro-termination attitude, we were apprehensive, and I was prepared for battle.

Almost as soon as we were led back into the ultrasound room, he came in. Before he could say one word, I told him, "We're keeping the baby."

"What about the other two?" he asked.

"They are no longer involved." I reiterated firmly, "We are keeping the baby." I made it clear that we would not tolerate discussion of termination. I was curt and direct. This matter was not on the table.

And to our amazement, Dr. Spencer changed into an entirely different doctor, charming and informative. He wrote down a link to the guidelines for ensuring that a baby with Down syndrome was getting the best and timeliest pediatric care.

Either this man is the moodiest dude I have ever met or one of his multiple personalities just appeared! Whichever it was, we were grateful, and I wasn't going to complain.

Dr. Spencer prepared Andréa for the scan as his assistant watched.

He turned the machine on and started to glide the wand over Andréa's stomach. We stared intensely at the large screen.

We immediately saw Delaney! She was alive and kicking. Right away, we both looked for the back of her neck.

I started to cry. Andréa started to cry. With tears in our eyes, we looked and winked at each other while we squeezed each other's hands. Before Dr. Spencer even said one word, we knew.

We could see it with our own eyes. The fluid was almost entirely gone! There was no cystic hygroma.

"Oh, my God, she's such a little fighter," I choked out, and kissed Andréa on the cheek. My already huge admiration for my new little daughter grew even bigger.

Andréa looked over at me. "She just wanted us to be her moms, Keston. That's all she needed," she said, as if we were completely alone in the room. It must have been quite some scene for Dr. Spencer and his assistant.

If we weren't already in love with Delaney before, we certainly were now! It was hard to stay composed throughout the rest of the exam. We were so proud of her.

I asked Dr. Spencer why he had written "cystic hygroma" on his initial report.

He just shrugged. "Well, that's a nonissue now."

Are you kidding me? While I knew Liz couldn't handle the Down syndrome, the words "cystic hygroma" carelessly included in the initial ultrasound report had definitely pushed her over the edge.

Because fifty percent of babies with Down syndrome have heart problems, Dr. Spencer referred us for an echocardiogram and scheduled repeat in-depth ultrasounds once a month.

We left that day with Delaney's first 3-D ultrasound pictures.

Andréa texted Erica and told her the news. She responded with a quick "That's great" and nothing else. We knew this had to be bitter-sweet for her.

We were on cloud nine as we drove home.

Delaney's First Photo Shoot

When we got home, Andréa posted Delaney's 3-D ultrasound photos on Facebook. I must admit the baby looked like an alien. But she was the cutest little alien we'd ever seen. She was holding her hands up as if to say, "I'm here and ready to fight."

We had a lot of encouraging comments on Facebook, but then we received a Facebook notice that Shawn had tagged himself in Delaney's photo. Andréa was taken aback. We didn't even know that they had accepted our friend requests.

Andréa promptly untagged him.

Within seconds, Shawn wrote a comment under the photo—"We need to talk"—for all of Andréa's friends and family to read.

Andréa deleted his comment.

"Panda, we need to email him," I told Andréa, and before she could say anything, I was on Facebook, messaging "Hi, Shawn, please feel free to call us," and left him Andréa's phone number.

Maybe they'll respond this time? These dudes were weird.

It wouldn't have surprised us if we'd never heard back from them. We were used to Shawn and Rod's brief bursts of communication, whether through Erica or in quick texts. We'd reply, only for them not to respond. They would disappear as if they had never communicated in the first place. So we weren't expecting it when the boys called that night. Andréa put the phone on speaker.

Shawn spoke first. "That picture floored me. It made everything real," he said.

Rod chimed in over Shawn: "We just want to make sure that we can still be uncles. We thought that maybe we could help you girls sometime, and take Delaney for a weekend every once in a while. It would give you a break."

Andréa and I were thrilled. Maybe they would be champions for our warrior as well! We promised to keep them in the loop.

The next day, I emailed them many links to our plan of action for Delaney, from the DSC advocacy groups to the therapies we had planned for her.

Then, just as abruptly as they had popped in, Shawn and Rod disappeared again.

Why were we not surprised?

Jared and Julianna Make It Simple!
February 11, 2013

It was a long, awful winter. I don't like winter anyway. It's depressing, and if the gloomy weather isn't bad enough, I really miss that extra hour we lose during Daylight Saving Time. This year, winter had been even harder for us than usual. We had been dealing with so much.

It was a welcome relief to see the hills turning back into their beautiful spring green. Everything was new, and the air started to smell of fresh foliage and flowers. It was our new beginning too, and our new little family member would be joining us soon. Andréa and I couldn't wait to meet her face to face. Jared and Julianna were starting to get excited too.

One afternoon, I realized that the kids had no idea what Down syndrome was. Andréa was on her way out to a Swiss Club meeting, leaving the kids with me.

"How can we explain it to them?" I asked her just before she left.

"Show them videos tonight for your 'Mommy-O and Me' date night," she suggested. "Show them the *Just Like You* video. It's easy to understand."

Just Like You was about three teenagers, who didn't have Down syndrome, talking about the disability and introducing their three best friends, who did have it. This video did a great job explaining in simple terms what Down syndrome meant, and what kids with it looked like.

As soon as Andréa had closed the door, I called the kids to sit with me and watch videos. With one of them snuggled up on either side of me, we watched the fifteen-minute film.

In typical Jared and Julianna fashion, as the video opened, the kids were more amused by tickling each other across my lap. I drew their attention back to the screen.

"This is what Delaney will be like." I pointed to a girl with the disability.

Julianna's brow went down. She pointed to another girl, the one who was narrating, who did not have Down syndrome. "And she'll be like this girl too?" she asked, as if she didn't want to believe what I was showing her.

I smiled and shook my head. "Nope, she's not like that girl."

Jared just watched the video and listened to us talk.

Soon another girl with Down syndrome appeared on the video. "Delaney will be like *that* girl too," I repeated and pointed to the screen.

Now both Jared and Julianna were totally engaged. They just stared at the screen without squirming or playing for the rest of the video. I could tell they were surprised to see what people with Down syndrome looked like.

It wasn't long before I looked over at Jared and saw he was wiping away tears. He was beginning to understand that his new baby sister was going to be different. This was not what he was expecting. It was shocking to him.

I wasn't quite sure that Julianna understood yet. She was still so little.

They didn't say one word while watching, but I did continue to point out that "this person has what Delaney has," and a few minutes later, "and this person doesn't."

Now they nodded. I thought at least Jared was beginning to understand.

When the video ended, I asked them if they had questions. Jared, who had been unusually quiet for the entire video, had many.

"Their eyes are weird," he said. "Is Delaney going to have weird eyes?"

"Yes, son, she will," I replied.

"Is she going to talk like that?" he asked.

"Yes, and she may not talk for a long time. That's why we're all learning sign language at dinner."

Julianna just listened intently to her big brother's questions and my answers.

"Are people going to be mean to her?" Jared continued.

"Yes, people have already been mean to her."

Jared, wiping away his tears, said fiercely, "I will protect her." And by the look on his seven-year-old face, I knew he meant it.

I bowed my head. "No, son, they're just being mean because they're scared. You have to let mean people know it's okay to be scared, but they should give your little sister a chance. Tell them that she's very sweet," I explained. I was too ashamed to tell him about my own fears that I had to overcome.

"But if they're still mean to her, I will beat them up," he insisted. Jared was going to be very protective.

Well, we'll cross that bridge when we get to it! I dropped the issue.

Julianna had only one thing to say: "Delaney will be silly."

"Yep, if she's like you, she probably will be, eh?" I agreed.

Sometimes the pureness in a child's heart makes everything so clear. We adults get so clouded by our own egos. We hide in imaginary boxes so no one can see what's truly in our hearts. We can't even see it ourselves. We're so worried about what other people are going to think of us. At first, I was terribly worried about what others would think of me if I were to have a baby with Down syndrome. My initial egotistical thought was *will people think there's something wrong with me?*

Jared and Julianna were free of their egos.

They didn't care that Delaney had Down syndrome. They had a "we'll be okay" and "we love her no matter what; nothing else needs to be said" attitude. It was just that simple for them.

Both the kids taught me a lot that day. They were genuinely surprised and sad that their new little sister would be different. From the looks on their faces, it was clear that this wasn't what they were expecting. But instead of being afraid, they were protective and proud. They were completely unwavering in their love and commitment to their new little sister. Everything was going to be okay.

I knew from that moment on that Jared would rise to every occasion to protect his baby sister throughout the rest of his life, and it reiterated what I already knew: Boppi was dead wrong about Jared! I was so proud of them.

They love Delaney no matter what! Hurray, Delaney has two more champions!

Getting to the Heart of the Matter
February 20, 2013

Over the next few weeks, Erica texted often to check in. She knew when the baby had appointments and always wished us luck. Even though I was sure she wanted reassurance that she'd made the right decision, my heart ached for her.

Dr. Spencer's office arranged for our pediatric cardiology appointment with Dr. Helton, who was upstairs in the same older building as Dr. Rose. His waiting room was large and painted orange. It was very cheerful and bright, and full of children's stools and books.

Dr. Helton came out to greet us himself. He was clean-cut, thin, and gray-haired, in his mid-sixties, mild-mannered, soft-spoken, and very kind.

He took us back to his ultrasound room, which was plain and dimly lit. A lovely multicolored papier-mâché butterfly hung from the ceiling for the children on the table to gaze at. On the wall at the head of the examination table hung a tie-dyed blanket with a peace sign. It was a quiet, soothing room. We relaxed a little.

Dr. Helton began Delaney's echocardiogram. This first time, he told us he thought she possibly had a small hole in her heart, as well as a leaky valve that he said was insignificant. She was still too little for him to be sure. He asked us to come back for a second echocardiogram when she had grown a little bigger. Once again, we would have to wait to find out how serious it was, but Dr. Helton was calm and reassuring.

The echocardiogram reminded us that Delaney did have Down syndrome, and she was going to have special needs. But Dr. Helton made us feel that even if there was a hole, it was small and might close up on its own. Everything could have been so much worse.

I remembered that even though we hadn't heard back from Shawn and Rod, we'd promised to keep them up-to-date on Delaney's health. I also promised Erica the same thing.

On the way home from Dr. Helton's, I asked Andréa to text Erica, Shawn, and Rod. Andréa quoted Dr. Helton's diagnosis to them: "The baby may have a hole in her heart and does have an insignificant leaky valve."

Erica's response was, "See, you never know what you're going to get."

Shawn and Rod had no idea the baby had even had a heart appointment. Rod didn't reply at all. Shawn replied, "What's a leaky valve?"

Andréa texted him a brief explanation and waited for his reply, which never came. More crickets!

Rod and Shawn either never responded to any of our communications, or Shawn returned an indifferent one-liner. We were getting used to it and really didn't pay it much attention. After all, they were only "uncles." We weren't expecting more from them. But why were they still keeping up the caring charade every once in a while? If we'd had the time and energy, we might have stayed more on top of it, but there simply wasn't any extra to devote to this slightly nagging question.

Dr. Spencer's About-Face
March 5, 2013

At our next ultrasound at twenty weeks, Dr. Spencer seemed pleasantly surprised Delaney was doing so well.

"Everything looks perfect. If I were to check her for the first time today, I would never guess she has Down syndrome," he said as he finished the ultrasound.

"She's in the fifty-sixth percentile in growth, which is unusual for babies with Down syndrome." He handed us a CD of pictures of Delaney's ultrasound.

Okay, I like this one of his personalities. Let's hope it sticks around, I thought.

Today Delaney could do no wrong in Dr. Spencer's eyes. Apparently, this little fighter didn't get the memo that she had Down syndrome!

On the way home we texted Erica, Shawn, and Rod.

Erica was puzzled. "So what does he say about the cystic hygroma?"

I was puzzled right back. Either Erica was testing me or she had memory problems.

"Erica, she never had cystic hygroma. We told you he said last time it was a nonissue." I was surprised she acted like we'd never told her before. Had she just not been able to take it in then? It felt more like she was almost accusing us of withholding this important fact from her.

"It was a big factor in our decision because of the added health issues and risks. He told us to terminate." Erica was upset with Dr. Spencer. "The CH was the scary part more than anything! The fact that the fucker diagnosed it, and it turned out not to be true, is bullshit!" Shawn replied to our text with his characteristic brevity: "That is great news. I look forward to meeting her." No questions. Nothing more.

Andréa and I raced home to see the pictures from the ultrasound CD on our computer. Delaney no longer looked like an alien. Now she looked like a perfect, adorable little baby. In one of the pictures, we could have sworn she was laughing! Later Erica texted me, "It was just a lot more than we expected, and then being told about the CH! We just keep telling ourselves that this little soul is obviously supposed to be yours and not ours! It is the only thing that gives us peace."

Chugging Along and Getting Bigger

Weeks were starting to turn into months. Every day the reality of this new little person was growing stronger. She and Andréa kept getting bigger. Delaney continued to be in the upper fiftieth percentile for fetal growth.

Andréa's morning sickness did not subside until mid-March. As soon as it passed, though, she knew what she had to do. Delaney needed to have weight on her side, so Andréa ate!

"Delaney craves chocolate," Andréa said with a crooked smile.

I laughed. "Oh, then you must give her what she wants."

Soon Andréa revealed to me, "Delaney also loves peanut butter. As a matter of fact, she loves peanut butter with chocolate." Hence, we started our weekly trips to Baskin-Robbins ice cream for Delaney's favorite Reese's peanut-butter parfaits.

Delaney was so active after Andréa's sugar highs that we felt like she was celebrating or maybe dancing to a feel-good song!

"I'm going to have such a hard time losing this weight later," Andréa said, but she was determined to gain it anyhow. "Delaney needs to continue to grow in case she has to come early," she reasoned. So she planned healthy meals along with the chocolate, and ate with intention.

Erica continued texting to ask how the baby was doing. When we told her good news, I felt she thought I was lying just to rub her nose in it. It was odd how I had to tell her again and again that the baby did not have cystic hygroma. She acted like it was new news every time.

"Don't you remember our long conversation about her not having it?" Can *she just not face this mistake?*

We had not heard from Shawn and Rod for weeks, but we saw on Facebook that they were going to the theater, to concerts, and took a trip to Hawaii! No wonder they didn't have time to be Delaney's "uncles." Still, after all that hoopla a couple of months before, we thought it odd that they never reached out to us.

"Maybe they never check in on Delaney out of some sort of loyalty to Liz and Erica," I suggested to Andréa.

"That's what I was thinking too," she agreed.

No Wedding on the Beach
March 22, 2013

We had everything in place now. Our little family had quite a few words memorized in sign language. Delaney would be here in no time!

One side of Julianna's bedroom became a nursery, even though Delaney would be sleeping with us during her first year. Instead of a crib, we got a convertible playpen. We let Julianna help us decorate. She picked out the colors: pink, pink, and more pink!

Most important, we were setting up Delaney's therapies. They could begin as early as when she was two weeks old, but more likely when she was three months old. There were four different therapies, and they were each approximately seven thousand a year. It was a huge relief to find out that we qualified for the fees to be waived. Delaney was going to have a chance to thrive!

My own life had changed drastically over the last few years. I had gone from being a regional sales manager to being unemployed—which I'm sure was a major concern for Tutu and Boppi. The job market had changed just as drastically as my life had; the types of positions I had held successfully for many years now required a bachelor's degree for me to even pass the first screening—which I didn't have. I found myself taking a part-time job in retail. I hadn't been in retail (or made this little money) since I was a teenager. I traded my tight-fitting, low-cut business suits and high heels for an orange apron and tennis shoes. And I found that I loved it! I had been a supervisor, manager, or high-pressure salesperson most of my working life. The no-stress pace, making friends, and helping customers all day long were a welcome relief. My part-time job turned into a full-time one, and I eventually took on a second job managing Toe-Rific Chocolates and Candies, a company that sells candy shaped like feet to savvy marketing managers and podiatrists.

Something dawned on me one night while I was lying in bed. "Hey, we haven't been invited to any parties in a long time," I said to Andréa. I was very aware that my inner circle had been decreasing, but now I realized our social life had almost come to a screeching halt. Andréa nodded, not paying much attention, while she played a game on her cell phone.

It wasn't long before I started seeing pictures on Facebook of my friends all having a great time at parties, holding up drinks and cheering at the cameras. "Hey, we were never even invited!" I complained to Andréa. I was deeply hurt.

"It's the kids," Andréa said, trying to make me feel better, but I knew that for the past two years, we'd always been known to get baby-sitters. Sure, we missed some parties, but not too many. Why were we off the invited lists?

I had to assess the situation honestly. My new life clashed with the lesbian party lifestyle. And now not only did I have small children, but I had a disabled baby on the way. No longer a queen bee, I had been ousted from the hive.

Well, at least I'll always have my loyal "outcasts," I thought. I mean, for goodness sake, I was the only one who'd stood by these castaways during heartbreaks and depressions. I had been the one inviting them to dinners and bringing them to parties so they could meet people. I was confident I would always have them.

But it wasn't long before the Facebook pictures of parties started including my outcasts. They were clearly now in with the "in" crowds, with the arms of the new queen bees—the ones who used to make fun of them—wrapped firmly around their shoulders. Only now, the outcasts were wearing makeup and had gotten rid of their face piercings. I realized that my absence from the parties and my vocal frustration over not getting invites made me the only common denominator among them; it gave these women the opportunity to make me the subject of exaggerated tales and gossip. It was bittersweet that I had introduced most of these people to one another.

I decided to stop torturing myself and quit going on Facebook. I knew I had a great life with or without superficial friends. And life was going on full steam ahead. Delaney was on her way!

Andréa and I were adamant about keeping Liz, Erica, Shawn, and Rod free of any legal responsibilities for Delaney. I would put my name on the baby's birth certificate, but in order for me to do that, we had to speed up our domestic partnership filing date.

Instead of having Andréa's small dream wedding on a beach after the baby was born, as we'd planned, we signed our papers in a notary's office. "Maybe we'll have that wedding once gay marriage passes," I said, trying to make her feel better. Andréa and I changed our names to Ott-Dahl. Delaney would be Delaney Skye Ott-Dahl.

We were starting to plan the baby shower and invited Liz, Erica, Shawn, and Rod. Shawn and Rod had made no effort to get to know us, so we thought this would be a great opportunity for us to make the effort. *Maybe one day they will reappear as uncles?*

During this time, Erica had texted me to ask how everyone was doing. I asked her about the baby shower.

"I'm not sure we'll come. We want to support you, but it might be too painful," she texted.

I understood.

I told her that Andréa and I had filed our domestic partnership so that I could put my name on Delaney's birth certificate, and she was going to have both our last names. I must have struck a nerve.

"You'd better check into that. I don't think you can do that," she texted.

I dismissed what she had said, but texted back appeasingly, "Thanks for the advice. I'll check."

About half an hour later, Andréa and I were sitting on the couch and writing up plans to rewire another room in our downstairs basement when her phone vibrated. She picked it up to see who had messaged her.

It was Shawn.

CHAPTER 14

Dancing to a Different Beat, but It's Still a Deadbeat!

"HOW STRANGE." ANDRÉA WAS PLEASANTLY SURPRISED.

She read his quick one-line text: "We need to talk."

By now we were used to this familiar line. But this time something didn't feel right.

I instantly had a sinking feeling. "Uh-oh, this means trouble."

Andréa waved her hand dismissively. "Nah, I'm not worried. They've been completely out of the picture. It's not like they want to be dads." She regarded Shawn's text as harmless. She shook her head and started imitating Rod's voice: "After all, they 'can't afford no babies,' remember?"

I still had a nagging feeling.

Then Andréa's phone buzzed again. Another text came from Shawn: "Can we talk now? We are just feeling more and more feelings for this baby, and would like to work out how we all can co-parent her."

The bombshell had dropped.

Andréa's eyes grew wild with anger and she started to spew, "Co-parent? Um, where the fuck have they been?" I was shocked to hear her cuss. She went from zero to sixty in the blink of an eye. "Do they not know the meaning of the words 'sperm donor'?"

I tried to calm her down. "Relax, Panda. Just tell them we need to think about it," I told her. "We need time to figure out how to deal with them."

She raised her eyebrows at me, her eyes still furious, but started typing a text back to Shawn with a speed to match her anger. She wrote, "Let me think about it. I really do not have any free time until Monday after Jared's baseball game."

Andréa's eyes were becoming wilder as the bombshell started to sink in. "How dare they treat Delaney like a whim! I would love for her to have father figures, but not deadbeats who rarely ever bother checking in," she stormed, her arms flying and fingers pointing in violent jerking motions. She was not giving me any time to react. "Delaney is not a novelty! Where were they in January, when the baby was fighting for her life? When we were being threatened with a lawsuit if we didn't terminate her?"

I tried again to soothe her. "Panda, relax. Maybe we could use the help. Maybe it's just more people to love Delaney." I got her to sit back down next to me on the couch.

Then another text came through from Shawn that added more fuel to the fire. She read it to me: "We wanted to give you a heads-up on where we're at. We want to be in her life as dads."

"Dads?" she yelled at the phone, and jumped right back up off the couch, where she swung around toward me. She couldn't contain herself.

I sat looking up at her. Before she could say another word, I calmly told her again, "Relax, Panda! Babe, I can understand why they would feel attached to that label. Who cares about a label?"

"They were never supposed to be dads!" Andréa's tone was sharp and nasty. "Deadbeat uncles I'm okay with. Had they wanted to be dads, they certainly shouldn't have acted like deadbeats. How about trying to get to know us? They could have gotten involved a long fucking time ago, and I would have been more than happy with them becoming dads,

but to this minute"—she paused and tried to gain some composure—
"to this minute, Keston, they have not asked once about Delaney: how
she's doing, if she needs anything...*nada*! The single person we ever
heard either of them mention any concern over is poor *Li-lo*." She
emphasized the name as if she were Rod speaking. Then she went back
to her own nasty tone: "Li-Lo this, Li-Lo that. Never once"—her finger
flew up in the air— "Delaney!"

Andréa's phone was still in her hand when it rang. It was Rod.

The Bulldozer!

"Answer it," I told Andréa.

She did and sat back down next to me on the couch. Once again she
became shy, but she was still angry.

I told Rod we were on speakerphone.

He was direct. "I read the texts between you and Shawn and thought
I'd better call right away. Shawn doesn't come across right."

"Okay...," I let him go on, expecting him to be less offensive than
his husband.

He was frank. "See, we aren't going to give up our rights. We've
decided we want to co-parent," Rod said sharply. I could almost picture
him on the other end of the phone with his hand on his hip as he laid
this thoughtless doozy on us.

Oh, okay, that was much smoother than Shawn! Not! *That was like a
bulldozer. And now I'm going to have to deal with Mama Bear*, I thought as I
looked over at Andréa, who had started to cry.

I wasn't mean, but I was direct: "Rod, your intent all along was to be
donors. We're going to have to think about this. This is shocking news to
us. I mean, you have to understand that we have to wonder where the hell
you've been. You guys don't call; you don't check in. You've never bothered to get to know us. Now you come to us out of the blue with this?"

He tried to talk over me, but I didn't let him; he needed to hear what
I had to say. "You have to understand what you're saying. What it will

mean to co-parent this baby. This baby already has her insurance and therapies set up. Now your incomes will come into play. Now you will both be subject to child support."

"Oh, no, we won't pay child support. We don't want all that. We'll just agree to pay for her when she's with us on our weekends."

Clearly, these idiots are oblivious to child support laws! I shook my head. "That's not how it works, Rod." I tried to make him understand the realities, but he bulldozed right over what I was saying.

"No, we will support her on the weekends we have her."

"Rod, we don't even know you two. We need to get to know you both," I interrupted. Perhaps you should come here, visit some weekends once Delaney is born? And we can start from there."

Rod plowed heedlessly on. "And we will expect that you do the same. We expect that half the time you'll be bringing Delaney to Gilroy to see us."

I remained calm as I watched the color in Andréa's face go from red to redder.

"Now, Rod, we have two other children who are in activities, and we'll be taking Delaney to four therapies a week. She's also going to be breastfeeding. She won't be able to do overnights until a doctor gives us the green light either way." I emphasized *either way.* "You will have to be considerate of these things."

Rod got snotty. "You see, that's exactly what I'm talking about. We don't want anyone telling us when we can and cannot see our daughter." He continued to talk as if he hadn't heard a word I said.

Andréa whispered angrily with her hand flailing, "'Our daughter'? She's not their daughter. They were fucking sperm donors who were to be uncles, and they've been shitty uncles at that." She was over-the-top upset.

I didn't see how this conversation could ever end, the way it was going. I had to stop it. "Look, Rod, we're going to have to think about all of this. We'll get back to you."

And with that I hung up. I took a deep breath and looked over at Andréa.

"I hate him," she said. "I just hate him."

I tried to make light of the situation. "Let's keep our fingers crossed that rotten Rod is not the biological donor." I thought about it. "They'll probably disappear like they always do, Panda."

Andréa stood up again and yelled at me, "Not before causing a lot of trouble for Delaney."

I don't think Shawn and Rod had actually ever given this idea much thought. It seemed like they were only acting on a whim. They certainly weren't caring about Delaney, or the effects of their freakish behavior on Delaney's mothers.

Honestly, considering they were gay (I'm sorry for my stereotype), I was a little surprised they weren't more touchy-feely and sensitive in their approach. At least Shawn had seemed to come off as more feeling and less "have it my way." We must have read him completely wrong, though.

Haven't these idiots ever had any women in their lives? Did they not learn from their mothers how they should approach us? Their selfishness shocked and disgusted me.

Andréa finally sat back down next to me on the couch, trying to digest Rod's demands.

I gave a deep sigh. "The timing is interesting. I can't help but think that Erica spun this. I mean, could these newfound 'fatherly feelings' have been intentionally or maybe even unintentionally instigated to punish us for Liz's breakdown?" I hesitated. "Maybe I've been talking about how happy we are just a little too much? Maybe I should have kept it quiet that I'm going to be listed as the other parent on Delaney's birth certificate?"

It wasn't such a far-fetched thought.

"I completely agree," Andréa muttered, while she was wiping away tears.

It seemed very likely that Erica was behind the scenes pulling strings, but in exactly what capacity, we weren't sure. I texted her, "Shawn and Rod are coming out of the blue wanting to co-parent."

Erica replied within seconds, as if she were waiting for my text. I read her response to Andréa.

"I think that they felt they didn't have a choice either, and now they feel since she is going to be here, they want to be a part of her life. You will have to work it out." I could almost hear her laughing.

They didn't have a choice either? Erica's use of the word *either* resonated in me. *Yes, Erica, you had a choice. You had the first choice.*

"The only choice Liz and Erica didn't have was to kill the baby," Andréa said. "We took that away from them."

What was left of our relationship with Erica started to unravel fast. But we still needed her as some sort of middleman. We now knew that everything we texted or said to her would get back to Shawn and Rod. We had to use that knowledge in our favor.

At this point Andréa had stopped talking. The look on her face was one of despair.

Their behavior gave us a clear picture of what the future with these idiots would be like. The problem was that they could really hurt Delaney, in more ways than one. They could jeopardize everything we'd set up for her.

"Look, who cares about the 'dad' title?" I pleaded with her. I understood the emotional attachment to that label, and I tried to sell that understanding to Andréa: "I didn't have a dad. It would have been great to have had a man in my life whom I could have called Dad," I explained. "Let's just get to know them. Maybe they're coming across wrong because they just really don't know how to properly establish themselves in our lives."

I felt terrible that Andréa had to go to a Swiss Club meeting in the city that night. She was in no shape for it. I had calmed her down some, but she was still deeply upset.

Apparently, on her drive home from the meeting, she stewed even more. It was late when Andréa returned. I was still awake waiting for her. With one quick glance when she came into the bedroom, I could tell my earlier calming effects had worn off. She must have been thinking about Rod's demands the whole way home from San Francisco.

She almost immediately started yelling—and she was loud: "I thought about it and *no*. I don't want to 'co-parent' with douchebags who have already shown that they're deadbeats. I don't need to"—she made angry quote gestures with her hands—'think about it.' They didn't ever feel it was necessary to call to check on Delaney when she was fighting for her life." She calmed slightly, still angry but no longer yelling, although she was getting more animated. "Delaney is not a novelty or a whim so that they can have their own baby shower."

Staring at Andréa with wide eyes, I whispered, "Shhhh...I know, Panda, I know. You're going to wake the kids."

"Or so they can be two gay dads, the heroes pushing their disabled daughter around in a stroller at Gay Pride parades!" Andréa's anger was escalating once more as she spoke. "Again, where the fuck have they been?"

"Quiet down, babe, shh," I said, but she didn't.

Shawn and Rod needed to make her feel better about them. It was the only way. If they were so ignorant of good behavior, I would try to educate them for their own sake.

Andréa finally went to sleep after her meltdown. I got up in the middle of the night and wrote Shawn and Rod an email. I didn't want interruption, denial, and reaction. I didn't want dialogue.

> Hey, guys, I am writing because I realize that you are new to all this, and you may be emotional. You may not understand or be aware that your abrupt approach is a hard pill to swallow. This was a shock to us. Up until now, you were only sperm donors who wanted to be occasional uncles. You have to understand that we have to ask ourselves, "Where the hell have you been?" I need Andréa to feel better about you. I need her to feel warm and fuzzy. We need to get to know you.
>
> You have not picked up the phone or texted once to ask about Delaney, not one time. That has to change if we are to work together. First and foremost, before you say anything to us, I need you both to ask how Delaney is doing. I need you to ask Andréa if she needs anything.

I need you to be respectful of our schedules, be considerate that we have other children, that Delaney will be breastfeeding, and that we will be driving her to multiple appointments every week.

You need to understand what this "co-parenting" idea entails. You *will be* financially responsible. What co-parenting entails for this child can have severe consequences for her.

Please think about what I am saying and your approach.

I sent it and blind-copied Andréa.

I hoped they would actually read the email. I hoped they would act more appropriately. I felt good about it. I smiled as I closed my computer and went to bed.

The very next night, Saturday, I received an email back from Shawn and Rod. We were at a dinner party with friends who were treating us to dinner for Andréa's birthday.

I thought this would be a positive response. I leaned over and read the email quietly in Andréa's ear.

"Hey, girls, obviously we need to talk. Please make time to have a phone conversation Sunday, as we feel this really needs to be addressed as soon as possible. We have nothing to gain except the love of *our* daughter."

I bit my upper lip.

Andréa closed her eyes and took a deep breath.

"Okay, 'our daughter' again? And didn't I just tell them yesterday that we have commitments and wouldn't be available until Monday?" she said. "So…?" she paused, twisting her fingers together and talking louder than I wanted her to: "They couldn't give a shit that we have commitments. We have to cater to their demands and call when they say? They didn't even read your email, Keston. I'm done with them."

I had tried, but Andréa was through. She was done dealing with these morons.

Andréa looked seriously at me. "They need to be fully aware of the entire situation. We need to be blunt." I knew she meant for *me* to make them fully aware, not *we*, as I let her continue. "And we're not going to call them when I told them we're not available."

The rest of the night was in shambles. We were not exactly in a celebrating mood. Later we lay in bed and talked about it. Andréa was resolved that she would have nothing more to do with Rod and Shawn.

Liz and Erica always went on and on about what great guys they were. In other contexts, they may have been. But not in this one.

I wondered aloud, "Why haven't we ever seen how great these guys are? I mean, not even in the beginning? They were never overly welcoming to us. They always treated us like we were outsiders. Shit, they never even offered us a glass of water when we were at their house!" To me, their behavior made no sense.

But Andréa finally smiled. Now that her rage had died down, she had it figured out at last. "Because Liz and Erica must have complained about the surrogacy monies. Shawn and Rod think I should have done a surrogacy without any compensation, strictly out of the goodness of my heart. They probably think I was in it for the money."

It was a mind-blowing thought, but I had to agree with her.

I got up in the middle of the night, because there was no way I could sleep after that horrible day. I went into the kitchen for a glass of water, thinking about our new dilemma.

I closed my eyes and channeled Mom. This was a time when I would definitely have asked her for advice. She could be ruthless. She would have given me valuable advice, which I would have listened to.

"Ma, what would you do?"

I smiled. I knew.

This was the instant in which Mom would have stopped being mad at me for choosing to have Delaney. She would have switched into protective mode with her grandma bear claws out.

Mom had zero tolerance for men who wanted to be sporadic part-time dads on their own whims. *"Ignore them,"* she said matter-of-factly. *"They will go away."*

"And if they don't, Ma?" I needed more of an answer.

With a wickedly raised eyebrow, Mom told me, *"Then bury them.*

Get an attorney, Keston, and bury them. They're bullies. They're cowards. Hit them where it hurts. They'll go away fast if you do."

Mom was a hundred percent right. I was absolutely sure of it.

You Can't Have Your Cake and Eat It Too
March 25, 2013

Needless to say, we didn't give in to Rod's bullying and demands to call them during our busy weekend with the kids. I took Mom's lead, and we ignored them. If they wanted to stew in their own juice, we were happy to let them. I thought about Mom's advice and I knew exactly what Shawn and Rod coveted most—Liz, and their bank accounts.

I would not have been at all surprised if they disappeared again.

But texts back and forth with Erica made me believe that she was still in the background, stirring the pot. This was going to be the last time I allowed her to do that. But I did use her machinations to our advantage up until that point.

I was at work the next Monday morning when my phone buzzed. It was a text from Andréa.

"Shawn sent me a text," she wrote. "He wants to know if we have time to call today?"

We agreed that we would call them that night after Jared's baseball game.

The day went on, and we went to Jared's game, came home, and got the kids settled in for the night. Then we decided to call Shawn and Rod. We were lying in bed when Andréa dialed Shawn's phone number and put the call on speaker.

She wanted me to be direct, so I got straight to the point: "You need to be fully aware of the ramifications—" I started.

Either Shawn or Rod snapped, "What's up? Get to the point."

That's what I thought I was doing. But I went on, taken aback by their now blatant rudeness. Whatever friendly tone they had had with us was now gone.

"Your demands with this child can have severe effects," I began, but was interrupted again.

"Get to the point." I believed it was Shawn who interrupted this time. It was hard to tell their similar voices apart.

I was surprised to hear Andréa throw in, "Look, no one knows if either of you are even her biological donor." She was hinting at the use of another anonymous donor. I looked over at her and squeezed her hand. She whispered to me, with her hand over the speaker, "If they want to be bulldozers, I'll give them a bulldozing dose of reality."

"You're a liar!" Shawn was obviously chomping at the bit. It was as if he had been dying to say that to us for months.

So much for his Mr. Great Guy image. This nastiness was only the beginning for Shawn and Rod. It was the first of many insults that started pouring out of their mouths. I won't repeat all the names they called us—mostly Andréa.

Clearly, these boys are spoiling for a fight!

The gates had opened. Shawn and Rod let all their pent-up resentment out. It was inappropriate and degrading. We had done nothing to them.

They both took turns bashing Andréa, mostly in indirect but obvious defense of Liz and Erica. Instead of fueling their fire, Andréa and I sat and let them vent. We let them dig themselves into a deeper hole.

"You're just greedy; all you want is money," one of them yelled. I believed it was Rod.

I was surprisingly calm, but still forceful as I rebuffed his attack: "Rod, usually surrogates are compensated. I can see how not compensating your surrogate worked for you two." I didn't want them to think they had shaken us.

But they had.

Andréa couldn't help herself. She spoke into the speaker, but, taking my lead, she had no angry inflection in her voice. "And because your surrogate backed out, now you want to take over Delaney? When right up to this minute, you still haven't even asked how she's doing? Delaney is not a puppy."

How Andréa maintained her cool I do not know. There they were, hurling low-blow insults at her, calling her horrible female epithets, and she stayed calm.

"You're a fraud," Shawn yelled.

"How am I a fraud?" Andréa asked quietly.

"You should give Liz and Erica back the money they gave you. You didn't give them a baby, did you?" *Bingo!* Shawn's voice sounded distant, as if he were leaving the room.

"I wasn't selling them a baby," Andréa defended herself.

I interrupted, trying in vain to put some clarity into their minds. "Andréa did more than she was supposed to for Liz and Erica. She went above and beyond when Liz and Erica didn't even pay her as they were supposed to." Shawn started spewing out dollar amounts that he felt Andréa and I needed to give back to Liz and Erica. It was very obvious that the two women were indeed behind this.

Andréa was more involved in this conversation than she'd intended. "You two were supposed to be uncles. You were sperm donors."

Rod retorted in a sharp tone, but I could tell he was now trying to match our calmness: "And, Andréa, so were you. You weren't supposed to be the baby's mother."

"That's true, but we were the ones who saved her life and then chose to be her mothers back in January. Where were you? And where have you been since then?" Andréa answered, as if she had expected his response.

I couldn't let them continue the attack. It wasn't easy for me to remain calm. *Do these morons not realize that Andréa and I have taken on a lifetime of financial responsibility? For the most part, taking the heat off all of them?* It really was too much to handle. I would take Mom's lead now, and I'd let them know I was going to hit them where it hurt.

I'd started to lose my temper, but I still didn't raise my voice.

Calmly I smiled and looked at Andréa as I spoke into the phone. "Rod, if you want to call us frauds, then by all means we will stop being frauds. We will put your name on the birth certificate and tell the State of California where they can collect child support for us." I paused as

I had a wicked thought. "And we will also tell them how the baby was created under a contract for your precious Liz and Erica as well. We will not be frauds, and we'll let the chips fall where they may. All four of you will be subject to paying child support."

I immediately felt bad for my nasty comeback, but not all that bad.

As if I had said the magic words, there was an immediate about-face. "Obviously we're not going to get along. We want nothing to do with you or the baby," Rod said truculently, to cover up his backing down.

Funny—the possible implication of money and their desire to protect Liz from exposure and child support was the end for them, at least for the time being.

"How do we sign away our rights?" Rod asked.

"In all honesty, we may not even have any control. I'll put my name on the birth certificate," I said, "but we cannot guarantee that this won't someday come back to haunt you."

Rod, in all his infinite wisdom, said in an exaggerated, over-the-top tone, "Trust me, we have a lot of money, honey; we'll get a good attorney and we will *never* pay a dime in child support."

What planet is this guy on? Isn't this a far cry from "We can't afford no babies; we only make fifty thousand a year between the both of us," which is what Erica said they'd said back in January?

"Yes, Rod, yes. You absolutely will be paying child support," I said without emotion. "Don't take my word for it. Ask an attorney."

Rod paused, and then blurted, "Then we'll just get custody of Delaney." He took another brief pause, "I mean, we might as well, right?"

Shawn was in the background yelling, "And we expect a call when the baby is born."

Rod spoke over him: "I don't care. I never want to see the baby." We heard them quietly arguing between themselves. Then Rod got back on with his last demand for us: "You need to call Shawn when the baby is being born. So he can see if she looks like him."

I shook my head in disbelief. "After how you've talked to us? We owe you nothing." I spoke flatly between gritted teeth.

"I mean, it'll be obvious if the baby is black, right?" Rod was sneering as he emphasized *black.*

Andréa confidently affirmed, "I can guarantee you the baby is not even remotely black."

"We owe you *nothing,*" I repeated.

"You aren't going to call?" Rod asked.

"We owe you nothing," I said one last time.

After the way they treated Andréa, the way they treated us—yelling, calling us names, not to mention the way they were missing in action when Delaney needed them most—why would they think that we'd call them when she's born? So they can stress Andréa out in the hospital? They're out of their fucking minds! Their ridiculousness astounded me.

"This conversation is over," I said emphatically. Rod agreed and we hung up.

Andréa and I looked at each other. I smiled a little faintly and said, "Well, that went over well." We were exhausted and bruised, but we'd gotten through it, and Rod and Shawn were backing off. The relief was overwhelming. Mom was right: We felt like it was over.

A few days later, I sent Rod and Shawn an email asking that they send me an original letter of intent from when they had donated their sperm, to protect them "just in case." Unsurprisingly, they ignored my email.

That was the day we learned that Erica had a bitterness inside her that was always going to rear its ugly head.

We had to say goodbye.

CHAPTER 15

That Damn Hole!

March 29, 2013

WE HAD THE SECOND ECHOCARDIOGRAM AT TWENTY-
two weeks and everything looked the same, although now Dr. Helton
was almost certain that Delaney had a hole in her heart. In his report,
he wrote, "Probable moderate VSD inlet hole."

When we got home, Andréa researched VSD inlet holes and read
that they rarely closed on their own. That was the first time we realized
that Delaney might have to have open-heart surgery at some point early
in her life.

Days turned into weeks.

At our twenty-eight-week ultrasound with Dr. Spencer, once the
technician started looking at Delaney's heart I could see the blood mixing
from one side to the other. I could actually see what looked like an opening
between the bottom chambers. Dr. Spencer came in and looked too.

He wasn't too concerned.

"This is to be expected. When will you be seeing Dr. Helton again?"

"In two weeks," Andréa answered.

For us, it would be a long two weeks.

Our worries were confirmed at our third and last echocardiogram with Dr. Helton at thirty weeks. This time, the hole was obvious to him as well, but at least the leaky valve was "minuscule" now.

"This baby will be having open-heart surgery. It's only a matter of when," Dr. Helton informed us, as if he were sorry.

We had already figured as much from what we saw at Dr. Spencer's. However, as prepared as we were, it still wasn't easy having our fears confirmed. On our drive over the Kirker Pass hill on our way home, we weren't talking as much as we usually did. We were too sad.

"If anyone can do this, it's Delaney Skye," I told Andréa.

Andréa didn't reply. She just looked over at me, biting her lip.

Our little warrior might have one last nasty fight ahead of her.

Ignorance Isn't Bliss!
March 31, 2013

I wish I could tell you everyone in the family was supportive of Andréa's and my decision to keep Delaney. They said they would of course support us. However, actions speak louder than words, and their actions were loud and clear.

Knowing my mom, I felt she would have come around by now, especially since I took her advice on how to deal with Shawn and Rod. Mom was very protective.

Boppi, Tutu, and Robin spoke volumes by ignoring the fact that Andréa was even pregnant. Tutu was much less obvious about it, simply because we didn't spend as much time with her as we did with Boppi and Robin.

Either we went together or Andréa went by herself to Swiss Club meetings and events with her dad and Robin. As she got bigger and bigger, they continued to ignore her pregnancy as if they didn't notice. Anytime someone approached Andréa to talk about her obvious pregnancy, both Boppi and Robin turned around and walked away. Boppi thought nothing of handing her heavy boxes of files to carry in and out of meetings, while Robin carried nothing.

Andréa came home from one Swiss Club dinner she had shared with them and was unusually quiet.

"What's wrong?" I asked.

After a few, "Nothing," responses, when clearly there was something wrong, Andréa told me, "I've always looked up to my dad. For the first time in my life, I'm ashamed of him." She tried to explain how he was making her feel: "He's always been a fair man, easygoing. And it's hard for me to see him acting cruel."

Before this, Boppi was her rock, and she'd felt like he could do no wrong. She knew this time he was wrong—dead wrong—but she couldn't bring herself to believe his heart was really turned against her and the baby. She tried to pin the blame elsewhere and make excuses for her father's rejection.

"I know Robin has never completely liked me. She thinks I'm spoiled. She likes me more now than she used to, but I think she's influencing him and maybe feels threatened. Sometimes, Boppi is easily manipulated by her. I love Robin, and she's a great grandma to Jared and Julianna, but she has a mean streak, Keston."

I reminded Andréa how mature she'd been earlier: "Like you said, he needs time. He'll come around." *I hoped!*

Still, we tried to function as normally as possible and not withdraw from Boppi. Andréa chose patience, but it was getting harder for her. Easter was coming, and we always went with Boppi to his chapter of the Swiss Club's Easter picnic. Andréa did not belong to this Swiss group. This would be a good opportunity for him to come around, but the holiday was approaching and Boppi hadn't yet asked us to go.

I kept asking Andréa, "Are we doing the Swiss Club Easter picnic? If not, let's plan something else for the kids."

"Boppi still hasn't invited us." Andréa wanted to wait a little longer. But they barely spoke now. It was just a few days before Easter when she got up the courage to call him and ask about the picnic.

He told her that if we would like to come to the festivities, we were to let him know and he would buy our breakfast tickets.

"See, maybe he just assumed we were going." Andréa smiled as if everything were right in the world again. I hoped she was correct.

Easter Sunday morning arrived. We parked and made our way to the table where Boppi, Robin, and some of Andréa's uncles and cousins were sitting. We started to greet Boppi and Robin, but as soon as he saw us, he got up and walked away, signaling to Jared to come with him.

From the moment we arrived, Boppi pretty much ignored Andréa and me. He spent most of his time playing with Jared and Julianna or socializing with other guests. It was almost as if Andréa and I weren't even there. Robin sat at our table and talked briefly with us, but only when the conversation pertained to Jared and Julianna.

By now Andréa was huge and obviously pregnant. People repeatedly approached our table to ask about her pregnancy, which seemed to be the cue for Robin to either change the subject or just get up and walk away.

When it was time to eat, Boppi finally did sit down at the table with us. There was no avoiding it. Our Eggs Benedict were being served! He made nervous small talk; he talked about our house, which he'd helped us obtain a loan for, and how the value had increased since Andréa and I had made all the upgrades and improvements. Eager for his approval and praise for the work we'd done, Andréa jumped right into the conversation, nodding and smiling as we talked about our achievements.

Robin got a mischievous smile on her face and looked at Boppi. "You know, we could rent it out for $1,800 a month now." Robin spoke snidely, as if she owned our house. Then she made a "get out" gesture toward us, throwing her thumb up over her shoulder. "We have some moving boxes for you." Boppi gave a big smile and laughed as if he thought Robin were clever instead of cruel.

Andréa and I looked at each other, and I could tell she was close to giving up on her father. I'd seen that look before when she gave up on Liz and Erica.

They had barely spoken to us all day, and when they did, this was what they had to say? Jokes about kicking us out of our own house, which we'd invested our entire life savings into? Andréa and I didn't think she was funny at all. Andréa was hurt, and I was insulted.

We ate quickly and then decided it was time to leave. We politely excused ourselves and gathered the kids to go. On our car ride home, Andréa didn't talk initially, but soon she started to vent.

"Not only did they completely ignore us and ignore Delaney, but they made jokes about kicking us out of our own house that we've spent well over twenty-five thousand dollars fixing up, not to mention the ten thousand dollars we put down and the money we continue to pay each month for the mortgage and insurance." She was at her wit's end.

I wished we'd never gone to this horrible Easter celebration. I didn't know what to say to her except to agree and let her talk.

"This is just not like my dad. I've never known him to be mean like this." Andréa looked out the window as I drove. "He'd better not take things out on Delaney. If he's mad at me, that's okay, but he'd better not be mean to her. That will be the deal breaker for me."

I was also protective of Delaney. "I know! After the way she's been treated now? And she'll already have too many mean fuckers of the world against her. It would be terrible if her own grandpa treated her badly or ignored her as well." I was with Andréa all the way.

"I'm going to call him," I was surprised to hear Andréa say next. Andréa's mama bear was helping her overcome her fear of confrontation.

Uh-oh! I was worried where their conversation might end up.

Andréa had to do what she thought was right. Unlike Liz, she'd grown a backbone. She was apprehensive about talking in general to people other than me, but when it came to her kids—and now especially Delaney—she had no problem standing up even to her parents. "He needs to know he's hurting me," she told me.

The next evening, she called Boppi. I gave them privacy. She was in the bedroom for more than half an hour.

I don't know what they said to each other, but I do know things gradually got better after that phone call. "He apologized," was all Andréa told me. I was grateful to hear it and didn't press for any further details.

Boppi wasn't going to change overnight, but slowly we felt like he started coming around; then he would revert. Accepting Delaney had to be on his own terms and in his own time.

Weeks later, at one of Jared's baseball games—Boppi came to almost all of them—I mentioned to him, "We're going to build a Doman track for the baby." Boppi didn't say anything, just listened. I explained that Doman tracks—like an indoor swing set with monkey bars—help babies with Down syndrome learn how to use motor skills.

The next Saturday, Boppi came to Jared's game. He and I sat together and watched. Andréa was at dance class with Julianna.

"I would like to build the kids a play set in your backyard. You know, with a slide and swings…and monkey bars," he explained in his heavy Swiss accent.

I couldn't help but smile.

Come Out, Come Out, Wherever You Are
April 2013

During another of Jared's baseball games, I noticed a group of kids playing on one of the fields opposite us. They looked different. "Is that a Down syndrome group?" I asked Andréa.

"I don't know." She was too absorbed in Jared's game to be interested.

"I'm going to find out." I got up to get a better look. I was on a mission. As I was briskly walking across the field, it dawned on me just how far I'd come.

Well, look at you now, Keston. Instead of leaving or looking the other way, here you are stalking these people! I laughed and shook my head at myself as I picked up the pace.

They were, in fact, a group of kids with Down syndrome. I watched them play baseball for a few minutes, and then introduced myself to one of the parents.

This was to happen again and again. I would notice and approach parents who had children with Down syndrome at the grocery store, at a county fair, or at my job. My family and I were now part of a new club. We met more and more families with children who had Down syndrome. Soon we were being invited for play dates, picnics, and outings. It was good for Jared and Julianna as well, as they started to become more familiar with Delaney's disability.

Lions, and Tigers, and Bears, Oh My!
May 31, 2013

As Delaney's due date was creeping up on us, both Andréa and I went through moments of fear.

Erica's "grab bag of unknowns" was rattling around in my head, as I tried to come to grips with it. And although we were hopeful, we were praying that Delaney wasn't biologically linked to rotten Rod. There was so much we couldn't know for certain until after Delaney was born. She could be born blind or with cataracts; she could have more severe medical problems than her heart; and she could have autism (which occurs in five to seven percent in those with Down syndrome which is substantially higher than the general population and an added scare since it runs in Andréa's family. I could not share these bursts of fear with Andréa though. She was bearing so much already. I didn't want to plant more seeds of doubt in her head or heart.

As I wrestled with these terrors, doing my best to handle them alone, I heard my mother's voice loud and clear: *"You get what you get. You will make the best of it, Keston."*

I didn't realize Andréa was having the same overwhelming fears, and, like me, was trying to hide them. One day I came home from work to find her sitting on the couch crying.

"What's wrong, Panda?" I asked her.

Her crying deepened and broken words came spilling out. "What if we're being overly optimistic, Keston? What if it's so much worse than we thought? What if my dad is right? He'll keep rubbing it in my face every time something more turns out to be wrong with Delaney. And we already know there will be things wrong with her. I can't tell my parents, because they'll say, 'I told you so. I told you so' all the time!' What is our life going to be like? Are people going to stare at us? Am I going to want to punch people in the face when they stare rudely at Delaney, Keston?"

Oh, God, this wasn't what I was expecting my first minute home. I hadn't even put my keys down yet.

I smiled, sat down next to Andréa, and held her hand. "I don't know, Panda. What we do know is that Delaney is a fighter, and she's never let us down before." I confessed my own fears to her: "I've been going through this too. Of course we're going to be scared, but we're all strong, especially Delaney. We'll get through this together."

We made it through our day of fear and went back to our fighting, optimistic selves.

Tutu's "Mama Bear" Saves the Day
June 1, 2013

The next day, Andréa took Julianna to her hula dance class, which she did with Tutu's halau dance group. Julianna loved getting to see Tutu every Saturday.

When they got home, Andréa was in a great mood. I found out why. She told me about the wonderful thing that had happened when Tutu came up to say hello.

Tutu had immediately noticed Andréa's red eyes from her meltdown the day before. Normally, Tutu wouldn't have said anything. But today she did.

"You look like you've been crying. What is wrong?"

Andréa was stunned. Tutu was such a private, reserved person who almost never opened up emotional conversations. Today was different. I could see happiness in Andréa's eyes as she continued telling me about her morning.

"My mom was too worried about me for her to wait and call later.

She wanted to know right then if I was okay," Andréa related to me with a happy smile. She was so moved—she'd been longing for Tutu to be close like this all her life. This morning Tutu had been willing to leave her comfort zone so she could meet Andréa's needs and show her support. This was huge in Andréa's eyes.

Andréa told her mother about her breakdown the day before, and how reality had hit her.

"Oh, I went through that a long time ago, the day I got your email," Tutu said. The two talked heart to heart. I'm not sure of all the details, but I do know how much better it made Andréa feel. Thanks to Tutu, Andréa and I had both weathered the storm. Those fears never came back again to haunt either of us.

Sometimes, there are things that only a mother can fix. Tutu's mama bear came out for Andréa and somehow made everything all right.

Another Delaney miracle! She brought her mom and Tutu close together, just what Andréa had always longed for. Delaney seemed to be saying, "Don't worry, Mom; there's good stuff in my grab bag too!"

Our daughter was making a difference already.

CHAPTER 16

Andréa's Scary Online July Club

BEFORE WE KNEW IT, SPRING HAD TURNED INTO summer again. Delaney was coming soon!

The hills were starting to turn brown, and it was already hot. Very hot. Our new-old house was even hotter inside than it was outside; 102 degrees outside felt like 108 inside. Andréa and I bought window mounted air conditioners, but they were no match for the heat. Of course, Andréa was carrying a toasty little furnace around inside her, and she was really feeling it.

When we'd gotten Delaney's diagnosis, Andréa had immediately joined an online group of women who all had babies diagnosed with Down syndrome. The group was called the DS Pregnancy Board. She also participated through the DS boards in a thread of women all due in July.

There were nine original members in the July Club. Two dropped off the boards within the first three months, and we had no idea what happened to them. By May, three other members had delivered stillborn babies. Those babies had had problems beyond Down syndrome, like failure to grow, very low birth weight, and extremely severe heart defects. There were now only four babies left in the July Club.

It was alarming.

"Delaney has weight on her side," we told each other optimistically. But we couldn't help but wonder just how bad the hole in her heart was. Would she be whisked away by helicopter to Oakland's Children's Hospital for immediate surgery the minute she was born? Would she make it to full term?

There was still a very real possibility that Delaney might not be born alive, that she would fail to thrive, or that her heart condition would be worse than we had thought. But our little fighter, with her already spunky personality, seemed to be up for the challenges.

Delaney was kicking up a storm in Andréa's belly. Her growth was still impressive, and she was as cute as a bug in a rug in her 3-D ultrasound photo shoots, which we got every month. In the 3-D pictures, Delaney seemed like the spitting image of her mother and her big brother Jared.

In our research, we had discovered that the chromosomal abnormalities of babies with Down syndrome are also present in the placenta. The placentas are prone to deteriorate early and cause fetal death or premature deliveries. Often doctors choose to induce delivery early for that reason.

I talked to Dr. Spencer about it at the next ultrasound. He agreed. "Yes, this does occur. But this baby seems to be doing fine. The placenta looks good."

He did offer to set up twice-weekly stress tests for Andréa, which is a test that monitors Delaney's heart rate and movement. "If she is starting to decline, we'll be able to tell," Dr. Spencer explained.

We breathed more easily after that. It was one more safeguard in place.

Don't Stress
June 6, 2013

We were glad we'd made the decision for Andréa and Delaney to participate in the stress tests. The baby passed the first couple weeks of testing. Everything was looking good, and it was encouraging.

Unfortunately, in the third week of testing, Delaney gradually became more difficult to wake up, and her heart rate didn't accelerate quite like it should. She seemed to be slowing down.

At our thirty-fourth-week ultrasound with Dr. Spencer, the tech looked puzzled as he was scanning Andréa's belly. "Oh, there she is," he said. He went and got Dr. Spencer, who hadn't yet come into the exam room.

Dr. Spencer picked up the ultrasound wand and slid it over Andréa's abdomen. "She's breech," he said. "So, are you ready?" he asked, as he began to try to manually turn Delaney around by pushing and pulling on Andréa's belly. It was very painful for Andréa.

"Ready for what?" she asked naïvely, while Dr. Spencer was still roughing her up.

"To deliver this baby," he told her.

"Well, in a month I'll be ready."

"I don't want the pregnancy to go past thirty-seven weeks. She'll be full term then," Dr. Spencer said as he continued to try to turn Delaney. This was the first time we found out that he didn't want Andréa to go the full forty weeks of pregnancy.

But Delaney was stubborn and wouldn't budge.

I don't blame her. I wouldn't exactly be a fan of Dr. Spencer either.

"Be prepared," he told Andréa. "And you should be prepared for the possibility of a C-section if she stays breech."

The idea was not something Andréa wanted to hear. She desperately did not want a C-section.

The clock was ticking, and we had to get Delaney to flip back into a head-down position soon. In typical Andréa-and-Keston fashion, we went to the Internet.

There were all sorts of home remedies and suggestions, from toe acupuncture to standing on one's head, burning herbs, and chiropractors. We opted for Andréa to try floating upside down in a pool. "It makes sense," I told her. The water would make the amniotic fluid more flexible, and being upside down would hopefully encourage Delaney to flip. That was the plan.

Luckily we had a friend, Joanne, who had a pool. Only she was out of town. Andréa texted her to ask whether we could use her pool in her absence, and she texted back right away, "Of course." We were headed out the door twenty minutes later.

The house was in an upscale neighborhood of mini-mansions. A neighbor let us know he was watching us when we parked in Joanne's driveway. I waved and yelled over, "We're friends. She offered her pool to us." I smiled, and he nodded.

The pool heater was broken, so it was difficult getting used to the chilly water, but after taking baby steps and shivering, Andréa and I finally were both completely submerged. We had a plan: With Andréa facing me, she would do a sort of sideways cartwheel, then I would hold her knees above the water, while she held mine below the water. But I kept sliding over toward the deep end, hopping up and down and trying to keep her knees and cute little tush in the air. Meanwhile, she was underwater and had wrapped her arms around my knees with her face in my crotch.

All of a sudden, massive bubbles began filling my shorts. Worried something was wrong, I pulled Andréa up as fast as I could. She flipped her wet hair out of her face but instead of drowning, she was laughing hysterically.

"What the hell?" I yelled at her.

She was still laughing. "The neighbors are all watching us from their second-story windows." She shook her wet head, laughing even harder. Her voice changed as she mimicked in an uptight, conservative-housewife voice, "'Crazy lesbians. Look what they're doing now.'"

Then I laughed too. "Yeah, this must look like some weird sexual thing. Well, it isn't working," I told Andréa.

Change of plan. This time, I would have Andréa facing away from me.

"Don't fart," I told her as she cartwheeled into the water.

Andréa immediately popped back up again. She was having a hard time holding her breath because she couldn't stop laughing.

"We have to get this done. Stop laughing!" I told her on one of her breaks for air. I was on a mission: Delaney must flip!

After many attempts, we still didn't feel the baby turn. "Stubborn little stinkpot," I said, amused because I knew she was going to need to be stubborn and never give up in her life.

We went home, mission unaccomplished.

The next day, Andréa decided to try again at Boppi's community pool. I was at work, so this time, she would be on her own. No one would be holding her feet in the air.

She told me later about her day. She swam upside down, doing handstands…anything. And all of a sudden, Delaney had gone crazy! "I think she flipped," Andréa told me over the phone, "but I'm not sure."

Delaney's baby shower was going to be in a week and a half. We hoped she wouldn't be attending in a different capacity!

Let's Do This!
June 20, 2013

At our next OB/GYN appointment, we talked to Dr. Rose about Dr. Spencer's desire to wait no longer than thirty-seven weeks. We also told him about the babies on Andréa's July message boards. Dr. Rose decided we should listen to Dr. Spencer's advice. "He's the expert," he said. "We tend to listen to the experts. She'll be full term at thirty-seven weeks, and this baby is big enough, so let's go ahead and plan this."

I saw Andréa's eyes well up. The shock of having this long, crazy journey almost over, in just a little over one week, was too much for her. But she quickly composed herself.

"Panda, we kind of knew she was coming early," I told her.

"At least she'll be coming after her baby shower," she agreed, wiping away her nervous tears so that Dr. Rose, who was still in the room, wouldn't see her nervousness.

We looked at our schedules and decided Andréa would be induced on July first.

We left Dr. Rose's office with nervous anticipation. Andréa texted her mom on the drive home, but she didn't call her dad.

"Why aren't you calling Boppi?" I asked. "You usually get on the phone with him first thing when there's big news." Her reason had never dawned on me.

Even though Boppi and Andréa had made some peace, she still had her doubts about him. "Every time I give him any news that isn't as planned or is bad about Delaney, he has a 'see, I told you so' attitude. And I just don't want it."

"This isn't an 'I told you so' moment. We had a feeling she could be coming early," I tried to reason with her. "It's normal for babies with DS. Are you sure you aren't just being sensitive?"

"No, he always does that now." She plainly didn't want to continue this conversation. "It doesn't matter," she said. "I'm not telling him."

Is Andréa right? Are all the naysayers going to judge our "bad decision" all the time?

This is going to be a long, hard road.

Celebrating Delaney!
June 22, 2013

I personally didn't want to spend money on a baby shower. "The money we're spending on the shower could be spent on Delaney," I told Andréa. But she insisted.

As many naysayers as there were around us, there were also so many wonderful people who came out of nowhere to donate baby items. Friends of friends slowly began hearing our story. We got used to coming home to find boxes of baby clothes, baby swings, and play centers left on our porch, sometimes with notes, sometimes anonymously.

By the time the baby shower was close, we honestly didn't need much.

But for Andréa, it was important to have as many people as possible excited and welcoming Delaney. "So many people are going to be down on her in her life. I don't want her life to start out that way. I want a celebration. A day just for her," she told me.

So, along with some great friends, we threw Delaney a very fun, coed, Hawaiian-themed baby shower at Joanne's house.

The day happened exactly as Andréa had dreamed it should. Everyone talked about Delaney, including Boppi, Robin, Tutu, and her husband Scott. That day she was not the eight-hundred-pound elephant in the room that everyone was ignoring. That day, Delaney's magic came through yet again.

Andréa's family members who hadn't seen one another in twenty years were brought together. Everyone celebrated. Tutu and Julianna performed an impromptu hula dance together, everyone loved the Hawaiian barbecue, and there was swimming, good music, and a lot of laughing.

Delaney—and her mother—were the real stars of the show!

Dr. Spencer, Mr. Hyde
June 27, 2013

Of course, I don't know what I was thinking. I had to have known that Dr. Spencer's Mr. Hyde couldn't possibly let us get through the rest of the pregnancy without freaking us out at least one more time. He had to give it one more "doom-and-gloom" college try.

As we were preparing for Delaney's arrival, Andréa had to go in for a final stress test and ultrasound to measure Delaney before her scheduled delivery date just four days away.

I was at work eagerly waiting to find out any new news about our baby girl. Andréa texted me, "Delaney looks great. She now weighs five pounds, twelve ounces. I wish you were here; she is so cute sucking her thumb. I haven't seen Dr. Spencer yet," she wrote. "I hear him outside the door."

I smiled as I read the text and got back to work.

Then all of a sudden, my phone was vibrating like crazy. "The baby's growth has stopped," I read in Andréa's text. Then another text popped up on my phone: "He might want to take the baby today."

"What?" I said out loud as I read the text. My coworkers looked over at me. My heart started pounding in my chest as I walked to the break room and waited for the next text.

"He said the reason we wait as long as possible to induce is to avoid time in the NICU [newborn intensive care unit]. 'This baby is going to the NICU no matter what,' he said. 'We might as well get her there alive.'"

"Oh, my God, we can't wait until Monday, as planned? He thinks her life is in jeopardy?" I texted Andréa back. "Let's get her out now."

I called her, and she answered on the first ring.

"I'm on my way," I told her as I was rushing to the time clock.

"No, Delaney and I are doing a stress test now. I'll call you back," she said, and we hung up.

We both should have known. Of course, in true fighting-Delaney style, she did great on her stress test.

Delaney sure does love showing up Dr. Spencer!

Andréa waited twenty minutes to talk to Dr. Spencer after the test. Finally, he came in to see her. He was very nonchalant, as if he had never mentioned getting Delaney out even earlier than we had already scheduled.

"Don't bother coming in for your NST on Monday morning. They'll monitor you at the hospital Monday night when they induce you," was all he said to Andréa. Again, the scare was a nonissue.

I wasn't sure whether I should be mad at Dr. Spencer or thankful that he made us be more realistic. But then again, I had to wonder how realistic he really was himself. It was hard to know with him.

We went through another very stressful weekend, thanks to Dr. Spencer, with all the unknowns swirling around in our heads one last time.

CHAPTER 17

Monday, Monday, So Good to Me

July 1, 2013

AT LAST THE DAY ARRIVED. THE INDUCTION WAS scheduled. We were to show up at John Muir at 7:00 p.m. on Monday, July 1st.

Dr. Rose had explained the procedure to us at our last appointment: "When you arrive you'll be given a cervix-ripening pill to start dilating your cervix. Then in the morning, hopefully you'll be ready for Pitocin. The process can take twenty-four hours after we give you the Pitocin. Delaney should be here by late Tuesday." He paused and waved his fingers as he was thinking. "Wednesday morning, maybe."

Wow, will she really actually be here?

Dr. Spencer's haunting words—"This baby is going to the NICU no matter what. We might as well get her there alive"—weighed heavily on our minds. Obviously, Dr. Spencer, who was considered one of the best perinatal doctors in the Bay Area, knew what he was talking about.

So how bad was it? Was there a chance Delaney would pass away? Could her heart withstand the delivery?

That Sunday night, I noticed Andréa had an odd, apprehensive look on her face as I took off my work clothes and lay down in bed. I could tell she was worrying about something, and I had a feeling I knew what it was.

"I hope I don't eat my words, Keston," she said as her lip started quivering. "The last thing I said to Rod was, 'I guarantee Delaney isn't black.' There's still a slim chance she's his. I just really hope that awful man is not the biological dad," she admitted.

Rod may not have meant to come off as the douchebag of the year, but he did it nevertheless. Andréa couldn't stand the man.

"I prayed about it," she told me. I was shocked. She didn't believe in God and refused to pray. I guess this was her one exception. Her praying spoke volumes to me about how deeply she felt about Rod. I didn't want her to be this stressed out, not now.

Like Andréa's promise in her last words to Rod, I now made that same promise to her—a promise that I knew I might not be able to keep: "Panda, I promise you Delaney isn't going to be Rod's. She's never let you down before, right?" I pleaded with her in a reassuring tone. "She has a special link with you, Andréa. She isn't going to let you down now. I promise."

"You can't promise that. It's out of Delaney's control. By the time I was her mom, she was already created." She knew I was making a silly promise, yet looked relieved, as if she wanted to have faith in me.

"I believe she's always been yours." I hesitated, and then went on. "Ours. She always knew. The only ones who didn't know at the time were you and I."

God, now I hope I'm not the one eating my words!

It was hard to get to sleep. We were like little kids on Christmas Eve waiting to wake up to see all the presents Santa Claus had left us. But eventually I drifted off to sleep and found myself waking up to the alarm on my cell phone.

I worked that morning. It felt almost impossible to get through the day. I was counting down the minutes until I could finally clock out, then go pick up my little family and get us to Walnut Creek for this huge event in our lives. We were incredibly nervous, incredibly excited, and scared to death.

At the baby shower, Boppi and Robin had volunteered to watch the kids the night of induction, and Tutu had offered to pick them up the next day and keep them until Friday.

On the drive over the Kirker Pass hill, I was trying to explain to Jared how traumatic being born could be for Delaney. "It's like being in a dark, warm bath, then all of a sudden being thrust onto a violent waterslide, only to be forced through a hole this big." I showed them by putting my index finger and thumb together.

"And Mama might die!" he blurted out.

Andréa and I quickly looked at each other. We were shocked to hear Jared say that.

"Well, that's unlikely. What makes you think that, Jared?" I managed to get out.

"Grossboppi told me," he answered without hesitation.

"Yes, but that's highly unlikely," I told Jared. Then, thank goodness, we got off-track and started talking about what *likely* and *unlikely* meant, and laws of averages and chances, and so on.

We dropped the kids off and were on our way. Funny! For a man who thought his daughter might die in childbirth, other than "See ya," Boppi didn't give Andréa a hug or even a "Good luck" when we left!

The hospital was only a few blocks away from Boppi's, so we were there in a matter of minutes.

The nurses checked Andréa in, and I handed them silicone bracelets I had made with, "Down syndrome Awareness" and "Luv 4 Delaney" printed on them. We wanted anyone who would be attending Delaney's birth to know that we were celebrating her and we were aware of her condition. I didn't want anyone looking at her or us with an "oh, no" look. I didn't want anyone to feel they had to give us bad news. I also told anyone and everyone we knew that Delaney had heart problems, so everyone needed to be prepared.

We were led to a birthing room that was state-of-the-art, but not so much so that it felt sterile. It was still a welcoming, warm room: very large, nicely decorated, with a balcony and a view. It was more like an upscale hotel room than a delivery room.

Andréa got into her gown and sat on the bed. We kept looking at each other, almost in disbelief that this day was really here. Let me tell you, I no longer had fingernails!

It wasn't long at all before a pretty blond lady came in. She introduced herself as Joy, Andréa's nurse.

Joy seemed frazzled and quickly apologized. She'd had a flat tire on her way to work. She had been on the freeway, and no one had stopped to help her. "So I might ask you questions more than once; I'm sorry," she told us. But she didn't; she was right on the ball.

Joy asked us what we were naming the baby. I told her, and explained that we already knew the baby had Down syndrome. Joy got a Delaney bracelet too.

She put two monitors over Andréa's belly: one to track her contractions and the other to monitor Delaney's heart rate. We immediately heard the familiar sound of our daughter's heartbeat.

Ta-ka-cha...ta-ka-cha...ta-ka-cha...ta-ka-cha.

It was music to our ears. "There's our little train that always can." I smiled with watery eyes at Andréa. It was a surreal, emotional moment.

Joy explained that anywhere she was in the hospital, she would be aware of what was happening in this room with Andréa and Delaney. Joy then got Andréa started on an IV. I held Andréa's other hand.

As Joy was putting in Andréa's IV, she explained, "We're going to ripen your cervix with a pill that I'll insert into your vagina." She paused while she stuck the needle into Andréa's wrist. Andréa winced and squeezed my hand tightly. "We'll start with one dose, and then every four hours give you another dose until you're ready. But if you haven't ripened by three doses, we'll have to schedule a C-section." She went on: "Hopefully by the morning, you'll be ripe enough to start the Pitocin. Then you'll go into labor, and you'll begin feeling your contractions. By tomorrow night little Delaney may be here."

Joy left to get the cervix-ripening meds. We waited.

About twenty minutes later, Joy came back in. "Delaney's heart rate dropped. We can't start the ripening meds until she stabilizes."

Andréa and I looked at each other, very concerned. For the next hour, we sat in silence listening to our little train.

Ta-ka-cha...ta-ka-cha...ta-ka-cha...ta-ka-cha.

"It's kind of appropriate," I told Andréa. "Delaney has always been the little train who could. She'll stabilize, Panda. She'll be fine." And right on cue, Delaney did just that!

Joy came back an hour later. Delaney's heart rate had stabilized enough to proceed. "But we'll have to keep an eye on her heart rate to see how she's taking the meds and the stress," she warned us. "After I give you the meds, we'll want you to sleep, so I'll give you a sleeping pill." Then Joy had me pull out a chair that folded down into an extremely uncomfortable bed, and I set it up next to Andréa so I could hold her hand.

We were running behind schedule, but everything was a go; the meds were inserted into Andréa's cervix, and we were on our way!

Is this really going to finally happen?

Andréa and I lay in the dimly lit birthing room, listening intently to our daughter's little heart and her fighting spirit. We tried, but we couldn't sleep.

Ta-ka-cha...ta-ka-cha...ta-ka-cha...ta-ka-cha was all either of us could focus on.

"Sounds like a disco song from a Swedish band in the Seventies," I told Andréa. Then I started to sing to the beat of Delaney's tough little drum, only I changed the words: "We soon will find / Delaney is one of a kind / Baby, she's the key / Welcome to the world, Delaney."

Andréa giggled, and for the first time since Thursday, when Dr. Spencer had made his NICU statement, we lightened up.

"I think this is really it, Panda," I told her. *We're going to finally get some answers and see what's inside that grab bag.*

Joy's work shift ended, and in came a lovely older African American woman named Nell. She got a bracelet too. She was someone who gave the impression that a big hug from her would make anything and everything bad go away. She was a delight. She talked about her philosophies of life; she called them "Nellisms."

"When you're my patient, you're my family," she said. I believed she meant it. Nell came in at 2:00 a.m. to check Andréa's cervix and prepare the second dose. Andréa was only at two centimeters, but her cervix was soft. Just as Nell was getting the second dose ready, she looked up at Andréa's monitor. "Hold on; I see contractions." She stared at the monitor for a few minutes. "Well, it looks like you might have only needed one dose. You're having early contractions, so I'll hold off on giving you the second dose."

We went back to sleep, or at least tried to. We were surprised that Nell saw contractions on the monitor. Andréa could not feel them at all.

I heard Nell come in a few more times over the next hours and work quietly in the dark. But I really couldn't sleep. I decided to go to the cafeteria to get a cup of coffee while Andréa slept.

Is He Taunting Me?

I made my long trek down the elevator, through long hall after long hall, each decorated with pictures or drawings of nearby Mount Diablo. I was the only person wandering the halls this early in the morning. I finally turned into the last long hall, where I could see the coffee machines in front of the cafeteria. I was almost to them when I noticed a large photo of a doctor on the wall. He had his hands upward and cupped together, as though he was explaining something.

Must be someone special, since this is the only photo of a doctor I've seen in this place.

I got my coffee and took a sip off the top to make it easier to carry on my trek back to Andréa. The coffee was surprisingly good. I turned around and started on my way when I glanced up at the doctor in the photo again. I stopped dead in my tracks.

It was none other than Dr. Spencer! I read the paragraph underneath his picture. It talked about how great he was and how he'd saved the lives of a set of twins. "Good thing they didn't have Down syndrome," I said out loud in the empty hallway.

I'll have to come back with a black marker to color in some of his teeth!

I was back in the room when Nell came in at 5:30 a.m. and woke Andréa up again to check her cervix. Andréa was now at three centimeters, so Nell decided it was time to start the Pitocin. "It could take twenty-four hours after this," Nell repeated what Dr. Rose had already told us. She continued. "But with any luck, it'll be sooner. After 9:00 a.m., Dr. Rose will come to break your water, and we can really get things going. Then you'll start feeling the contractions," Nell told us as she was administering the Pitocin.

Oh, my God, was luck on our side!

Almost immediately, Andréa started to feel contractions coming on strong enough to hurt. She was still adamant that she would have a natural birth without pain relief.

At 6:00 a.m., Nell introduced her coworker Jackie, who was taking over. Nell's shift was ending, and we were sad to see her leave.

Jackie was a middle-aged woman with dark hair pulled back in a ponytail. She wore black eyeliner with heavy bright-blue eye shadow. We didn't get a chance to talk to her much, as she was busy taking over Nell's patients.

What's the Big Rush, Delaney?
July 2, 2013

Jackie finally reappeared around 8:30 a.m.. to check Andréa's cervix. Andréa was at six centimeters, and everything was moving in the right direction. Jackie offered her pain meds.

By now, Andréa's contractions were uncomfortable enough that she'd stopped talking, but she refused any pain relief.

"Babe, are you sure you don't want any meds?" I asked her.

"I don't want them." She sounded annoyed that I'd asked.

As soon as Jackie left the room, Andréa asked me to take her to the bathroom. I had literally just taken her right before Jackie came in. "You just went. But okay," I said as I unhooked Andréa's monitors and grabbed her IV. I held her arm as she waddled into the bathroom, where she sat down on the toilet.

I waited to hear her pee, but nothing was coming out. Instead, she gasped. "I have to wait to pee. Oh, no, I'm having a *bad* contraction!"

Telling her to breathe, I stood in front of her and massaged her back while she leaned into me, squeezing me tightly around my waist.

"It's over," she finally said, panting in relief.

"Okay, Panda, go pee now and let's get you back to bed."

But Andréa still just sat there. I heard no trickling as she stared at the floor. "I want pain meds." She waved her hand at me, and then put it quickly back onto her knee.

I left to find Jackie.

As I expected, Jackie hadn't gotten far. I found her sitting at a desk right outside Andréa's door. "She's changed her mind and wants the pain meds."

Jackie looked up from her computer, nodded, and got up. "No problem. I'll be in right away." She was on it.

I came back and Andréa was still on the toilet. She told me that she hadn't peed yet. For the third time I told her, "Okay, Panda, pee now and let's get you back to bed." But Andréa still either couldn't or wouldn't go.

I felt a hand on my shoulder from behind. It was Jackie. She looked over my shoulder at Andréa. "I have your meds, honey," she said.

"Panda, let's forget peeing. Let's get you back to bed so you can take your meds. I'll bring you a bedpan if you need it," I tried to coax her. But she wasn't budging.

"Oh, God!" Andréa yelled. "Another contraction." Then, urgently: "I am having this baby right now!"

Jackie smiled at me and then reassured Andréa, "Honey, I just checked you and you're only at six centimeters. You have a long day ahead of you. Let's get you back to bed and I'll give you your pain meds. Dr. Rose will be here in just a minute to break your water," Jackie insisted, and Andréa nodded in agreement.

The three of us waddled slowly back with Andréa and helped her get into bed.

Jackie decided to humor her. "While I have you in this position, let me just check you again." She quickly slid on a pair of latex gloves and leaned down to begin her examination.

The unconcerned look on Jackie's face changed and she gasped. "There's the baby's head." She literally turned around and ran out of the room.

Wait! What just happened? What does she mean, "There's the baby's head"? Where is the baby's head? And where did Jackie go?

Within seconds, Jackie was back in the room, but this time she had an entourage of people following her. I looked around in shock. People were flipping on lights.

We have hours to go, right? I felt the heat of the baby's bassinet being lit up and prepped behind me.

Andréa lay there, oblivious to all that was happening in the room. Moaning and shaking her head back and forth with her eyes closed, she yelled, "I've got to push."

"No, don't push yet. Dr. Rose is downstairs and he's on his way up," Jackie tried to calmly tell Andréa. All the people were moving around very fast. I had no idea what they were doing.

The next contraction was coming. "I want to push!" Andréa yelled again. Jackie put the palm of her hand flat against Andréa's vagina. She told Andréa, "Do not push. Dr. Rose should be here in a minute."

Andréa only shook her head back and forth, but then nodded, acknowledging that she understood.

I looked down and, to my shock and horror, saw Delaney's head up to her nose protruding! The baby was still in her amniotic sac, and Jackie was holding her in. "Oh, my God, Panda, I see Delaney's head!"

"What about the water? Can she be born in her water sac?" I asked Jackie.

"Yes, it'll be fine." Jackie didn't bother to look up at me as she nodded. She was trying to get Andréa to focus on something other than pushing. "Look, it's your baby's head," she exclaimed to Andréa to distract her.

"I don't care," Andréa yelled back.

Just then Dr. Rose came bustling in. Nurses were already standing at the door holding up his gown. He ran in and thrust his arms right into the gown. The nurses followed behind tying him up on his way to Andréa's bed.

He arrived just in time to catch Delaney by the shoulders. Once she was mostly out, he cut a hole in the amniotic sac by her neck and out emerged our little Delaney.

She cried immediately, and I cried too.

Our Warrior Emerges

"Do you want to cut the cord?" Dr. Rose asked me.

Before I could answer, Andréa, who hadn't spoken much at all during these last twenty minutes, popped her head up and quickly answered him: "Yes, I want her to cut the cord."

Dr. Rose handed me what looked like a normal, everyday pair of scissors and showed me where to cut, and with one snip, for the first time, Delaney was on her own!

The nurses whisked her over to the heated bassinet and immediately began checking her over. I was still in shock and was watching as I held Andréa's hand. We heard the nurses talking about Delaney: "Wow, look at all that fair hair," one said loudly.

Andréa heard it too. She looked up. She had just remembered her prayer.

"What do you mean, 'fair hair'?" I called over to the nurses.

"It's unusual for us to see a newborn with such long blonde hair," the head pediatrician replied.

I got the biggest smile on my face. My promise came true. I leaned over to whisper in Andréa's ear, "Delaney has blonde hair. I told you." She knew what I meant.

The head pediatrician who was working on Delaney summoned me. "You can come over and hold your daughter's hand." I later found out her name was Dr. Birk-Aetna. She was a petite and pretty blonde.

I looked at Andréa, who nodded at me, and I went to see my new little daughter up close for the first time.

Delaney was beautiful. She didn't have an extra head or sixteen toes. To my amazement, she was absolutely lovely in every way. I put my index finger in the palm of her hand and she grabbed it tightly, as if she never wanted to let it go.

It astounded me. I didn't expect her to be able to do that yet. I knew from my research on Down syndrome that her motor skills might be slow in developing, but here was our little warrior firmly gripping my finger. Tears of pride and adoration streamed down my face. I couldn't take my eyes off Delaney Skye. She was simply amazing.

I went back to Andréa, who was being worked on by Dr. Rose. Dr. Birk-Aetna was whispering to another doctor, and the two kept putting their stethoscopes over Delaney's chest. I knew they were listening to her heart and consulting each other about it.

Uh-oh, this is it! I was preparing myself for bad news.

Dr. Birk-Aetna came up to me. "What exactly were you told is wrong with Delaney's heart?"

I loved how all the doctors and nurses called Delaney by her name. I don't remember any of them ever calling her "the baby." I explained what we knew about the VSD inlet hole.

"Well, we don't hear anything." She saw the look on my face, and then quickly clarified, "Meaning I do not hear a murmur. To me her heart sounds fine."

Stunned, I asked Dr. Birk-Aetna, "Can I go with Delaney to the NICU?"

She gestured no with her hand. "Delaney won't need to go to the NICU." She beamed.

What? But Dr. Spencer was so sure she would.

Dr. Birk-Aetna added, "We'll keep an eye on her, but I see no reason for her to go to the NICU. We will keep her here in the hospital for forty-eight hours, but I believe she should be going home with you after that."

Holy shit, you have to be kidding me! I should have known! I looked over at Delaney, smiled, and nodded. As soon as Dr. Birk-Aetna turned around to talk to a nurse, I went up to Delaney, leaned over, and kissed her forehead. "You amaze me. Mommy-O loves you so."

I told Andréa what was happening. We just looked at each other with admiration, pride, and elation.

Let Me Call You Sweetheart...

It wasn't long at all before we were moved to a well-baby room, meaning a normal maternity hospital room. As soon as we were alone, Andréa and I sat in the hospital bed holding our new, wonderful daughter, and gazing at her in complete awe.

She was small, but ridiculously cute. "She's perfect. We couldn't have asked for a more perfect daughter," I cried.

Soon a nurse came in to take Delaney for a bath. I went too. In no time, we were back in Andréa's room. Andréa was talking on the phone. Delaney was in her bassinet, and I leaned over her, entranced.

I felt a presence in the room that by now was all too familiar. I closed my eyes, then opened them and said silently, *"Hi, Mom."*

She was standing on the other side of the bassinet inspecting her new granddaughter. Without looking up at me, she said matter-of-factly, nodding as if she'd known it all along, *"She's beautiful. She's perfect,"* in an "I told you so" tone. Mom was funny that way.

And I smiled with tears in my eyes. *"Yes, Mom, you're right."*

Eventually, a nurse came in to get Delaney for her heart scan. I didn't want our daughter to be alone, so they let me come hold her tiny little hand while she went to the nursery and underwent an echocardiogram. We needed to see what was really going on with her heart condition. It would take hours to get the results.

Back in Andréa's room, we were eager to see what color Delaney's eyes were, but she barely opened them, and only for very short squints.

"We have plenty of time to see her beautiful eyes," Andréa told me.

The first visitors who showed up to see Delaney were Tutu and

Scott. Tutu was completely enamored with her grandbaby. I know it meant a lot to Andréa to see her mother clearly won over by our little underdog's fighting charm. "Open your eyes," Tutu kept whispering in Delaney's ear, but Delaney wouldn't.

Next came Boppi, Robin, Jared, and Julianna, and our room became a party. Boppi came over and scooped Delaney up without saying much of anything to anyone else. He held Delaney, scrutinizing her, for a very long time. He couldn't take his eyes off her. He studied her toes and held her hand, he smiled intently down at his granddaughter, and when it came time to leave, he didn't seem to want to give her up. I could see he was wearing his Delaney bracelet.

Delaney had won over her grandfather's heart.

Finally, everyone left. Andréa and I once again sat together on her small bed, and I was holding Delaney. I started to sing to her the song I had sung to her so many times before.

"Let me call you sweetheart / I'm in love with Delaney Skye...," Delaney started to open her eyes and was blinking. "Let me hear you whisper / that you love Mommy-O too."

Now Delaney opened her eyes wide for the first time and looked right up at me.

She recognizes my voice; she knows the song. I started to cry and couldn't keep singing. I saw teardrops falling from Andréa's nose. She said while crying, "Finish the song, babe."

"I can't," I choked out, as tears poured down my face.

But I tried.

"Let me call you sweetheart / I'm in love with Delaney!"

The Monster in the Mirror

YOU KNOW, YOU GET UP IN THE MORNING, YOU LOOK in the mirror, and you think you know the person who's staring back at you. I was as confident about myself as being a caring, thoughtful person as anyone could be. I knew I had a fear of disabled people, but I didn't ever consider that I was a bigot. Because I was a friend of the friendless and because I took care of people, I thought I was just a great person. I never thought the way I treated disabled people or the fact that I was repulsed by them might be considered prejudice, but it absolutely was. In this, I was extremely unkind.

But I had been given a second chance by an amazing little muse. She gave me a unique experience, a bizarre divine intervention that made me look in that mirror, and I was shocked at the monster staring back at me. Me…this great person?

Had the circumstances not been different—my guilt for my role in Mom's death, my love for Andréa, our long journey trying to help Liz and Erica, and my ultimate falling in love with Delaney, the little warrior—I am certain I would have made the same decisions as Liz and

Erica. I wouldn't have been able to do any better. Our little warrior is the amazing gift that I have been given. She made me see that I could do better.

Andréa and I now know what I believe Delaney always had planned: We were always meant to be her mothers, from the very beginning. We used to say, "In our next life, we'll have babies together." With my age, and already having the responsibility of two small kids, we would have never had a baby together in this life. We certainly weren't going to accidentally get pregnant.

But the stars lined up, and a perfect storm happened. Delaney chose us. It had to be under these crazy conditions, because in any other situation, she would not have been ours.

Andréa and I think about Liz and Erica a lot. They are not the bad guys. I could have easily made the same decisions. I can imagine their pain. It was agonizing rereading the four-hundred-plus pages of transcribed texts and emails, even the happy and funny parts, that we documented for this memoir. We knew ahead what the outcome would be for Liz and Erica.

We wonder how they're doing, especially Erica. Did they ever become mothers? We hope they have. We hope their dreams have come true.

I also think that if they opened their eyes and saw Delaney today, if they were one of her many blog or Facebook followers, they would have a chance to have a change of heart, forgive themselves (as I forgave myself), and rid themselves of any guilt they may or may not have. They still can do better too. It is never too late.

Delaney Today

Delaney has never once ceased to amaze anyone and everyone with whom she comes in contact. As we are closing this book, she is two years old; she still has blonde hair, is insanely adorable, and has the most contagious smile! She is and always has been small for her age.

She did in fact have serious heart problems, but they were fixed by a wonderful surgeon and the amazing staff at Children's Hospital in Oakland when she was three months old.

What has been remarkable is that, developmentally, Delaney is either on schedule with or sometimes ahead of other babies her age, and I'm talking about children without her disability! We feel that early intervention and the choline Andréa took during her pregnancy contributed to Delaney's advancements. Cognitively, she is like any other two-year-old, she takes direction, knows when she has been naughty, gets mad, and loves to please. Delaney signs around fifty words and can verbalize what she wants. She giggles, plays with dolls, and absolutely *loves* to dance and sing, even though we have no idea what words she is making up. Sometimes, she babbles on, as if what she has to say is seriously important. Many of those times, I believe she sees and is talking to my mother, her grandma. She's a real charmer.

Everyday, Delaney is doing things that she isn't supposed to be able to do because of Down syndrome. We are a pioneering family because of our early start in Delaney's preventive care, which we document in blogs and on Facebook. We demonstrate a day-in-the-life of what Down syndrome looks like when babies are given early intervention; it is a game changer for them. I now know that such children are amazing gifts to society.

Today, I am so proud of my little family, of myself…of Delaney. The world is a better place with her in it, and her many gifts to her fans, friends, and society have only just begun.

I have become a Down syndrome awareness activist, living my life to change misconceptions about Down syndrome, hoping to open the eyes of people; those who are like the person I used to be.

When Jules told me how sad she was after watching Frozen because "there are no princesses like Delaney" and how she and Delaney could never be like Anna and Elsa. I realized she was right.

Growing up in Anaheim and being a loyal and lifelong Disney fan, I realized who better to be a hero for children of all abilities than Disney, but I am just one voice. It is with the hopes of reaching one thousand signatures, Andrea and I started a Care2 Petition to gather our plea to the Mighty Mouse.

We reached our thousand signatures in one hour and, to our amazement and surprise, the petition gained support from all over the world and as of the printing of this book has almost 100,000 signatures.

SPECIAL THANKS TO SPECIAL PEOPLE

Liz and Erica. We would not have Delaney today had we not embarked on this crazy journey with you.

Maryanne Williams. Luckily for me, I always had the sounding board of my dear friend Maryanne. We have been friends for twelve years. She was really there for both Andréa and me during this time, with wisdom and grace. I would have really been lost without you, pal.

Jan Wright. For encouraging me to write this book.

The Down Syndrome Connection, Bay Area. For being there!

All the women on Andréa's Down syndrome message boards.